EATING
UPSIDE
DOWN

GO VEGAN FOR HEALTH AND WEIGHT LOSS

BELINDA BUTLER

The information contained in this book is based on the research and personal experience of the author. It is not intended as a substitute for consulting your own physician. Always check with your medical doctor before making any changes based on information in this book.

ISBN: 978-1-4834-0363-2 (sc)
ISBN: 978-1-4834-0485-1 (e)

Library of Congress Control Number: 2019909702

Lulu Publishing Services rev. date: 10/08/2019

CONTENTS

PREFACE

Right at the start I would like to make clear that I am not a medical doctor, but I know from the experience of losing 94kg (207lb)– that's more than half of my original 164kg (362lb) body weight - that I have a story many people might want to hear about and learn from.

There's a lot of conflicting information out there in nutrition land. It seems that for every piece of advice that tells you to do one thing, there's another that says the complete and utter opposite! What's a mere mortal to do?

I happened upon the solution to my morbid obesity by chance. All of my life I have been fat. For the 30 years up to 2009 I followed the official health guidelines as exemplified by the food pyramid. My weight skyrocketed into the stratosphere and my health took a near-fatal dive to the deepest depths. I finally took fate into my own hands: I turned the guidelines upside down and transformed my physical and mental health beyond recognition. Really! It regularly happens that people I have known for years just don't recognise me any more.

This is me aged 48 weighing in at 164kg (362lb).

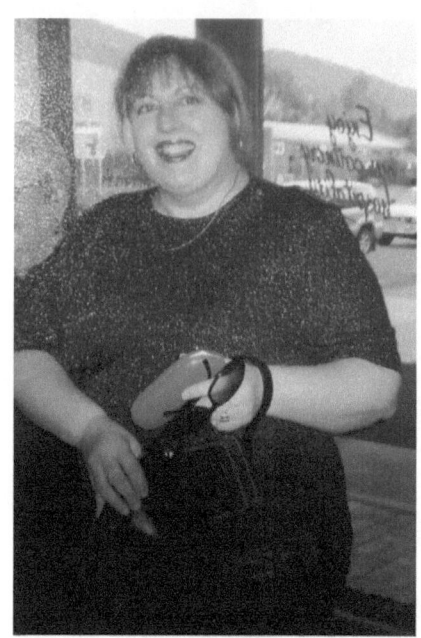

The author at 164kg (362lb).

And this is me now:

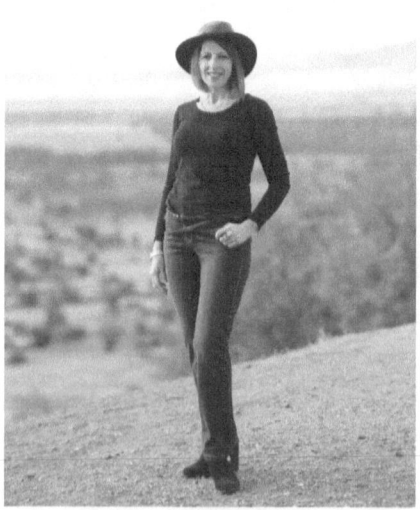

The author now at 70 kg (154lb)

My metamorphosis began in 2009 when I was diagnosed with type 2 diabetes. Later that year my mother nearly died from a dissecting aorta – a heritable condition that had killed her father at age 63 and which also claimed the life of her brother.

The well-meaning souls at the local diabetic clinic advised me to follow the official nutritional guidelines: eat plenty of whole grain foods and low fat everything else. Since that exact advice had damn near killed me I ignored it and did the opposite. I chose to eat a plant-based diet, low in processed foods in an effort to lower my blood sugar levels and avoid my family's vascular Achilles' heel. I dubbed my diet low-GI vegan. It worked.

I found I could eat to my heart's content and still lose weight. I have never felt deprived or ill; in fact my health couldn't be better! (Touch wood!) My body used to be 48% fat, now it's 16%. My triglyceride levels, and every other blood serum measure, were totally out of whack - now they're exemplary. I took a slew of medications that cost a fortune and which had hideous side effects: my medicine cabinet is now empty.

How and why did this happen? There was no magic pill, just an enjoyable and sustainable lifestyle that brought freedom from bullying, freedom to let loose and enjoy life and, most important of all, extreme good health.

Being a scientifically curious type of person, I decided to undertake research in this area to discover how and why this way of living worked for me. A plant-based lifestyle isn't for everyone, but some of the changes I made may work for you or someone you care for, too. The science is clear. Check it out.

Belinda Butler
Tamworth NSW
April 2017

INTRODUCTION

WHAT IS LOW-GI VEGANISM?

One of the main things I've learned along my path from 164kg (362lb) to 70kg (154lb) is how to deal with being the brunt of vegan jokes! But the joke is on those who continue to eat themselves to death. Instead of letting their old eating habits die hard, they choose to zoom down the highway to nutritional Armageddon and die-hard themselves.

So what is this thing I call low-GI veganism? Well, let's start with veganism itself: is it just another diet or is it an entire lifestyle, and more to the point, is it too much trouble to bother? The answer to the first question depends on why you choose veganism, although in essence it is characterised by not consuming any form of animal products.

Is it too much trouble? Well, that depends on whether you think your current lifestyle is really working for you. If you keep on doing what you're doing, will you be healthy and active into old age? Or are you destined for a life full of chronic pain? Will you be bed-ridden due to the complications of type 2 diabetes, with rotting limbs and a dialysis machine for company? Will you develop any number of autoimmune diseases that are afflicting more and more people? Making positive changes to your eating habits is the cornerstone to manifesting the health and weight loss changes you want. Are you truly happy with the way things are going for you, or do you want, or need, to make a change?

Some people choose veganism for health reasons, in which case it could just be a diet like any other. Some of these people, like me, find that it becomes more than just a diet, that it is a sustainable and enjoyable way of living. I believe this factor has contributed to my success in a big way. Others choose veganism for ethical reasons: cruelty to animals being a high priority. Sometimes people become vegans for both reasons. I became vegetarian at age 18 for ethical reasons, but even now, the more I learn about the conditions of farmed animals and the production of animal products, the more convinced I am that veganism is the right thing for me. It's kind to me, to animals and to the planet.

As for low-GI, what's the point of choosing a vegan lifestyle for its health benefits and then continuing to eat processed and sugary foods that have a high Glycaemic Index (GI)? That might be fine if you're only vegan for activism's sake but if you care about your health then a processed vegan diet is as bad as any other diet full of processed foods. Supermarket shelves are groaning under the weight of the many unhealthy, processed vegan foods that are now available. Such foods tend to have a high GI, which means that they will rapidly convert to glucose in your body once eaten. The higher the GI score, the more quickly the food converts to glucose, leaving you in a lethargic sugar coma until you get your next hit. Eating lots of high-GI foods can impair glucose metabolism and be a leading cause of weight gain and diabetes. Such a diet can really stuff you around. Although GI is not the only measure to go by when trying to choose healthy foods, it certainly helps.

Your body might object to your initial efforts to follow a low-GI vegan regime, but for reasons that will become clear in this book, your taste buds and your gut microbe buddies will soon come to adjust to your choices and love you for taking a load off their microbial shoulders.

Once you've got the hang of this low-GI vegan gig it is actually very simple. Choosing healthy food options becomes second nature after a very short time. Basically, if you have to read a label to know what's in a product, then it's not a good choice. This is not to say that you have to cut out all fast foods, snacks and pre-prepared meals, but keep them for manic days and special treats. To help seekers in their quest for health my Eating Upside Down blog is loaded with info, ideas, tips, tricks and hacks to make low-GI vegan simple and enjoyable.

HEALTH CONSIDERATIONS

Recent research uses ever-more sophisticated techniques to reveal how a lot of what we thought we knew to be true about nutrition is just plain wrong. From the 1950s onward the role of gut health was trampled on by scientists and corporations chasing down the golden goose of nutritional science: the ultimate weight loss pill. More recently some mavericks quit the chase and turned their attention to a non-pharmaceutical approach to optimal health. It turns out that the lowly gut and its microbial microcosm are absolutely crucial to weight control and our physical and mental health.

Once gut research got traction and a modicum of respect within the scientific community it was shown that antibiotics, once the saviours of mankind, have a dark side and can undeniably be considered an insidious scourge. They hide their toxicity behind a cloak of medical benevolence. Of course they have their place in the front row of the medical arsenal and they continue to save millions of lives every year; the problem is that they are also an underlying cause of many more diseases. Up until recently this was not recognised or admitted to by the medical community at large, but with the advent of more sophisticated scanning and research techniques it has been shown that antibiotic use can contribute to many so-called lifestyle diseases like type 2 diabetes, IBS, autism and certain mental health problems. This will be discussed in Chapter 6.

Man may think he can play God, but he just doesn't have the same finesse. He has tried to take a leaf out of the Great Maker's book by attempting to outwit and improve on nature, only to bungle the job so badly that he needs to seek atonement. Since the end of World War II there has been a proliferation of chemicals in our environment: they're in our food, in our household items and in pretty much every aspect of our lives. They're in the clothes we wear, the cosmetics we use, the food we put in our mouths and the utensils we use for cooking: all these things are laden with artificial substances that harm our health, making us tired, depressed and obese. None of these things come alone to the party. They inevitably bring along some other, uninvited guests. This is not good news. We need a miracle. Fortunately that miracle is in the offing.

ETHICAL CONSIDERATIONS

People around the world have come to believe that Western lifestyles, as exemplified by Americans and Europeans, are the epitome of success. Look at what I can afford! Eating meat, and plenty of it, is a sign that you've made it, that you can afford to be at the top of the food chain. An ever-increasing demand for meat and animal-based products on the international market means that more and more animals have to be raised and slaughtered to meet that demand.

The sheer volume of meat desired by an expanding human population means that traditional practices of farming animals out on the open range, allowing them to eat natural grass is virtually a thing of the past. Few countries are able to maintain these practices to any satisfactory degree. The vast majority of animals raised for human consumption are held in stalls or on feedlots. Animals living in such crowded conditions contract diseases and to treat these diseases we poison their systems with antibiotics and chemicals. I have already highlighted the problem with these so I use the term poison intentionally. It's time to take a step back and have a good look at what we're doing. Are we headed in the right direction, or have we taken an off ramp to nutritional oblivion?

WHY THIS BOOK?

This book is a recount of why I became a low-GI vegan and the profound and lasting effects it has had on me and my health. In early 2009 before I changed my lifestyle, I weighed 164kg. To look at me, you would have thought all I did all day was sit on a couch and eat: that I scoffed whole cartons of ice cream in a single sitting and that I never put one foot after another on a pavement. The truth was completely different. I was always health conscious and followed the official dietary guidelines and the food pyramid to the letter: I'm very conscientious like that. Since I was 18 I had tried to do a good 30 minutes of reasonably strenuous walking every day – also recommended. When I lived in Germany and Sweden I exercised even more. I also believed that the authorities who produced the food pyramid and nutritional guidelines were experts on the subject. I was wrong. They too, were led astray.

A friend's father who was a kindly local GP in my hometown once told me, "It's not the bread you eat, it's what you put on it." I swallowed every last letter of the low-fat gospel, thinking that I was doing the right thing, even though all the evidence veritably screamed to the contrary. Each letter of that advice was a health bomb waiting to explode. All you had to do was look at me to see that the advice wasn't working. I looked like the food pyramid I was following.

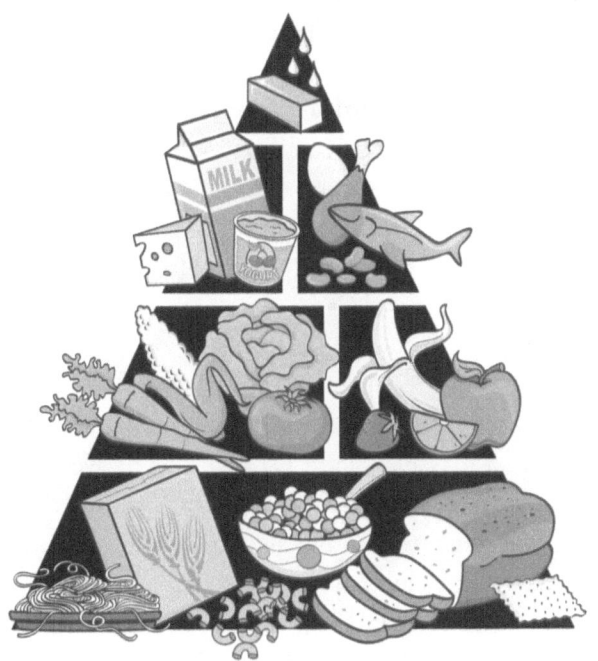

The Healthy Eating Pyramid 1982

For a vegan, looking at the food pyramid is like trying to play "Where's Wally?" You have to examine it very carefully to spot the one leafy green depicted on the diagram. What is easy to spot are the large chunks of pyramidal real estate devoted to animal-based and grain-based foods. (Yes, grains are plants but they come with caveats). In my opinion, the only thing right about this pyramid is the sugar at the apex. I left it where it rightfully belonged, but overhauled the rest. Following official dietary advice put me at death's door.

Twin studies across the globe reveal that genetics isn't everything when it comes to determining our health and longevity: environment and the foods we eat have a hell of a lot to answer for when it comes to switching genes on and off. But as genetics is important, I will tell you a little about my family and my history.

Mum always fought a losing battle with her weight, my brother as a child had rolls of fat, I had a massive gut and dad, although not fat, was not small either and that was largely down to the fact that he did a lot of physical graft on the farm and did daily calisthenics as well.

Mum had a penchant for all things savoury and although she proclaimed to all and sundry that she wasn't inclined to eat sweets, she was never far from a ready supply of crackers and bread. What she never realized was that these savoury foods harbour as much simple carbohydrate as sweets and they pack just as big a metabolic punch. Needless to say we developed eating habits akin to mum's – lots of processed carbs but also, thankfully, lots of vegetables.

In 1988 I was diagnosed by a local GP with pervasive candida and was given capsules and a massively long list of foods to avoid in order to kill off the pervasive yeast infection. I was told that candida thrived on wheat and yeast and that I must strenuously avoid these things. I managed it. Rye sourdough bread was delicious, but I had to give up my lifelong vegemite habit. A month or so after starting the anti-candida regime I moved to Germany to take up a German government (DAAD) scholarship to do my PhD. The stress of moving country and doing post-grad research meant I failed to complete the regime, and that failure has recently come back to haunt me – more of that later.

In my first year at Münster I needed to go to the gynaecologist a few times for unexplained shooting pains in my abdomen. The doctor said nothing was wrong and that it was probably because I wasn't keeping warm enough – being an Australian in a cold climate. In the summer of 1989 I went to Sweden for a Swedish summer school but despite the balmy summer warmth the pains returned. When I got back to Germany I rang my gynaecologist, but being summer, he was away on holiday, so I got in touch with another specialist.

Fortunately I got an appointment within a couple of days, and it was the change of doctor and his rapid intervention that saved my life. My new doctor gave me an ultrasound and then immediately packed me off to hospital that same afternoon for an emergency operation: left any longer the fist-sized cyst in my left ovary would highly likely have burst and that would have been the end of me. Up to that stage I had never heard of polycystic ovaries before, and in the pre-internet world there was virtually no literature available for me to find out more. The hospital doctors told me that no one really knew what caused it or the endometriosis that accompanied it. I now know that Polycystic Ovarian Syndrome, or PCOS as it's more commonly known, can be tied to the metabolic trap that had ensnared me and which led to much more dire health consequences for me.

Over the years I became fatter and fatter with every day that went by. I strenuously held myself to the food pyramid and government eating guidelines, reasoning that even if I was fat, I must be at least be healthy because I was doing "the right thing". The low-fat diet made sense: eat fat, you get fat. I avoided fat like the plague. Knowing what I know now about the dangers of low cholesterol and super low-fat eating I just pray that some of the insidious consequences of the long-term, very low-fat, high processed carb diet haven't already set themselves in motion somewhere deep inside me (MS, Parkinson's, Alzheimer's and the like). I am hoping and praying that eating a low-GI vegan diet with good fats may have turned around the worst consequences of my former polyunsaturated lifestyle full of grain/seed oils and carbohydrates processed to within a nanometre of their existence.

Meanwhile, thanks to that government-prescribed lifestyle, my blood sugar levels had been creeping up and up, hovering in the pre-diabetic range for many years. My GP asked me what I was doing about my weight. I listed off the exercise and all the healthy foods I was having based on the food pyramid guidelines and the sensible portions I was eating: whole grain bread, polyunsaturated oils like sunflower seed oil, low-fat margarine, low-fat yoghurt, low-fat cheese – if it was marketed as low-fat then I believed it was good for me. So did my doctor. She couldn't understand why I was putting on so much weight, why my triglyceride values were climbing along with my blood sugar levels. In 2009 the inevitable happened: I was diagnosed with type 2 diabetes.

MY FOOT ON THE LADDER TO GOOD HEALTH

Crazy how it takes a crisis to summon the momentum to seek change. After the initial realisation set in I managed to overcome my stunned inertia and bought a slew of books off the internet and most of them echoed the advice given to me by the diabetes educator at the hospital clinic: eat plenty of quality whole-grain products (65% of my calories), keep to a low-fat diet (use seed oils, and eat low-fat dairy) and exercise at least half and hour per day. I immediately saw that what these people had to offer was nonsense. Following such advice was exactly how I had eaten my way into this predicament in the first place. However, one of the books I had bought was different – it suggested eating a vegan diet. I wasn't prepared to do that, despite many years as a vegetarian.

It was my second wake-up call in 2009 that made me look seriously at changing to a vegan diet: my mother, who had several stents for aneurysms, suffered a dissecting aorta. For those unfamiliar with this diagnosis it means that her main blood vessel, the aorta, split apart and instead of blood being shunted around the body through her veins and arteries she was bleeding to death internally. A brilliant surgeon in Sydney actually saved her life and she only passed away less than a year ago. But the same disease profile had taken her father's life at age 63 and more recently it took her brother's. It ran in the family. My brother and I were advised to have scans every couple of years to detect any onset of these particular vascular problems. More research on vascular health convinced me that a vegan diet and lifestyle could be the solution. Something had to change. So I gave it a shot.

Looking back, I now know that it was a combination of following the low-fat, higher-carb mantra, chemical overload (environmental as well as medications for PCOS and depression) stress and genetics that caused the harm and made me grossly obese. Funnily enough, the one thing that has stayed constant is the way I exercise and the amount of exercise I do. Let me tell you, if you're obese, and you need to lose obscene amounts of weight, don't expect exercise to help you, not even if you put in hour upon hour of hard graft each and every day. And who, other than professional athletes or reality TV weight loss contestants, has time for that? If you have work and family commitments that's just not practical, or really useful. In fact, studies have shown that strenuous exercise during the weight loss phase of a reduction regime is counter-productive.

WHAT I KNOW FOR SURE

There is one thing I know for absolute sure, and the reason for it will become obvious as you read on: a calorie is not a calorie and what you put in your mouth matters a hell of a lot more than the amount of exercise you do when you're trying to lose weight (once the weight's off that paradigm changes, but we'll talk more about that in a later chapter). There's a whole lot of science on why low-GI veganism worked for me. It may sound odd, but it freed me from the cravings and psychological dependence on foods that ushered me to the threshold of metabolic oblivion. How the gut affects mental health is also fascinating.

WHAT'S IN STORE FOR YOU IN THIS BOOK

In the coming chapters I will explain how the foods we eat determines the gut microbes we have (the microbiota). Too many bad microbes can lead to a cascade of problems that slippery slide you to ill health, physical and mental misery and the supercilious condemnation of society at large: after all, it's OK to be rude about the fat person because they brought their hideous condition on themselves, right? Well, as you will see, this is often just NOT the case.

A lot of the most recent research into health and nutrition has yielded results that fly in the face of received wisdom from fifty years ago when Ancel Keyes, the "fat-is-bad" mogul, bullied his ideology into mainstream acceptance. Flawed, and sometimes unethical science paid for by big pharma and big food companies made the "fat is bad" mantra into dogma and ruined the lives of millions of people worldwide. If you're one of those millions of people, or know someone who is, read on and find out why obesity has become an epidemic and what can be done about it, especially if it's a personal battle for you. I can highly recommend Nina Teicholz' thoroughly researched "The Big Fat Surprise" if you are interested in the nitty gritty of this topic.

You won't find a prescriptive diet appended to this book, but you will find a list of resources for you to check out at your leisure. Some are links to online information and blogs, while others are books and articles for you to pursue your interest in any of the topics raised here. You can also read my blog called 'Eating Upside Down'.

Remember: there are certain principles that hold true for most human beings. However, everybody's body is different. What works for one person, may not work for another. Try whatever takes your fancy first. Experiment. Find the right path for you. Be open to new knowledge as it comes along. Don't look back, though, because that's not the way you're going!

CHAPTER 1

YOUR HEALTHY GUT

THE SILENT PARTNER THAT MAKES ALL THE IMPORTANT DECISIONS

Want some cutting edge science to really get your teeth into? Nutrition is where it's at. Gut health in particular. Great advances in medical science have come about in these fields and there is a plethora of literature available to the layman and the scientist alike.

What you put in your mouth has consequences way beyond mere satiety and enjoyment. Your food is your medicine. It determines most of what happens to the physical and mental health of you and your descendants. Yes, you read that right: what *you* eat helps determine the physical and mental health of your children and your children's children.

Nutrition is the latest science to break through the layers of accepted scientific dogma into a brave new world that overturns previous paradigms and ideologies. The most ironic thing about modern advances in this area is that "everything old is new again". It may be back to basics as far as the actual food is concerned, but the understanding of *why* we need to return to eating unadulterated, unprocessed, clean foods is now coming into focus with ever increasing clarity.

Ten years ago, if you had been searching for information on the causes of obesity, mental health disorders, Irritable Bowel Syndrome or thyroid disease you would have found scant research that pointed in the direction of the lowly gut: it was all "eat a low-fat, high-carb diet and exercise like crazy". But with each new piece of research comes the realisation that most of that advice wrong: the crucial missing piece of the puzzle was gut health. The condition of the gut is critical to so many aspects of health and it certainly paved the way to ill health for me.

Over two thousand years ago in ancient Greece, Hippocrates said that, "All disease begins in the gut". However, the medical community mummified this notion and laid it to rest until quite recently when interest in gut health had a magnificent revival. New discoveries are turning so much of what we thought we knew on its head. New findings continually fly in the face of what has become perceived wisdom over the last fifty years or so. It has got people in the field excited but there is proving to be a huge lag time in it filtering through to the practitioners at the coal face of daily medical practice: such is the extent and staying power of the toxic fat-makes-you-fat mantra. Lifelong indoctrination into the low fat syllabus of nutrition makes it hard to adopt a new perspective. It can take a fair bit of convincing evidence and research to wedge open the door to a brighter, newer, healthier world.

MAINSTREAM MEDICINE AND ADVICE THAT KILLS

Your average GP, diabetes clinicians and many health journalists, continue to advocate the low fat, high carb approach as a solution to our most pressing health problems; obesity, type 2 diabetes, thyroid dysfunction and the plethora of auto-immune diseases amongst them. Even the Diabetes Association of Australia continues to advocate the low fat, high carb regime. As of April 2017 this is what Diabetes Australia recommends on its web site:

"Grain foods such as breads, cereals, rice and pasta

Grain foods should make up the majority of our diet, so try to eat these foods at every meal. Go for wholegrain varieties, like multigrain bread, wherever possible to make sure you get long lasting energy and plenty of fibre.

The grain foods group includes foods like:

- breads
- breakfast cereal
- oats
- rice
- pasta
- noodles
- crispbreads
- crumpets
- polenta
- cous cous
- quinoa

Often people are concerned about eating too many foods from this group, particularly if they are trying to lose weight. But these foods tend to be very low in fat and will keep you fuller longer, particularly if you choose wholegrain options."
(April 2017)

This advice is no doubt well meant, and is based on the food pyramid, but if you follow it slavishly as I did, you will only exacerbate your condition – your health will only get worse. Contrary to the official claims, a diet based on the food pyramid is not a healthy diet. As you will discover in a later chapter, the types and amounts of food recommended will not "keep you fuller for longer" – fat does that - and fats are greatly restricted if you follow official dietary guidelines. You will, however, crave your next fix of carbs just like any other addict craves their poison. You'll also get the extra calories that come along with that. Eating a diet based on the food pyramid will put you on a merry go round that goes faster and faster, making it harder and harder for you to get off and find real nutritional solace in a healthy whole food plant-based diet – what I call a low-GI vegan diet.

RESEARCHING THE INVISIBLE – Microbes galore

A quick overview of what the latest research in the field of nutrition tells us can only whet your appetite for more knowledge about this topic, and if you suffer from one or more of the modern-day diseases, like I did, it may give you hope and inspiration for the future of your health and the health of the ones you love.

Gut health strongly impacts mental and brain health, obesity, inflammatory diseases, vascular health and immunity – especially autoimmune disorders. We'll discover that pretty much all so-called 'modern' diseases stem from dysfunction of the gut.

Our gut is full of microbes and when all is good in microbe-world we are usually in peachy health. Just by being a modern person, leading a normal modern lifestyle and making normal daily decisions about what to eat and how to respond to our environment continually impairs the functioning of the gut. This leaves us vulnerable to diseases that were once rare, but which now afflict an ever-growing number of people.

It is common to attribute diseases like Alzheimer's, Parkinson's, and MS to ageing – and there is a certain correlation - but losing your mind and mobility do not have to be inevitable companions of old age. By following a predominantly plant-based diet, we can shuffle them off to languish on the sidelines of life, while we get on with a fuller more active life ourselves. A lot of the damage that leads to these diseases starts very early on in life from the compound effects of poor diet, stress and trauma, medications and environmental factors all of which negatively impact the health of our guts. The human body is a finely tuned organism with checks and balances for every process. Although our bodies tolerate many of the terrible things we subject them to, there is only so much that can be done to repair the damage we inflict on ourselves. But it can be done.

Because our digestive tract, from mouth to anus, is the interface between us and the outer world, the things we eat, feel and experience directly impact it. As the human population grows, life gets harder; we have to use chemicals to grow sufficient food and provide enough clothing, time is a commodity in short supply leaving us rushed and stressed. As a consequence many of us suffer from what is called a 'leaky gut' and as we will discover, it and its causes are at the root of most modern-day diseases.

YOU'VE SPRUNG A LEAK - What is a leaky gut and how does it get that way?

Although I was diagnosed with Leaky Gut in 2003, I dismissed the diagnosis because it seemed so vague and inconsequential compared to other things happening in my life at the time. I should have paid more attention – a lot more attention. Leaky Gut is a term that we are beginning to hear more frequently. It develops when a variety of factors such as food allergy or intolerance, stress, trauma, medications and an imbalance of gut microbes cause the gut lining to become permeable. Having holes in the gut lining allows uninvited molecules to cross from the outside of the body (whatever is in your gut is technically outside your body) into the bloodstream where they can cause inflammation. Study after study shows that inflammation is the basis of most degenerative diseases.

Leaky Gut and its associated complications have been implicated in a slew of modern day diseases such as asthma and allergies, arthritis, autoimmune diseases, autism, mental health disorders and of course, gut problems such as Irritable Bowel Syndrome and Crohn's Disease.

How can we tell if we have it? Sometimes you can have a leaky gut and have no noticeable symptoms until something more sinister like MS turns up. Mostly however, we can tell because an array of nuisance complaints will surface. Taken individually some of the complaints in the following list may be mundane, everyday occurrences, but when they come together in a cluster and start to cause a general feeling of malaise, then it's time to take a closer look. Have you experienced any combinations of these symptoms on more than a short-term basis?

- Chronic (on-going) joint pain
- Chronic muscle pain
- Difficulty concentrating
- Bloating and digestive problems
- Changeable mood and depression
- Anxiety
- Acne
- Eczema and Psoriasis
- Poor immunity (e.g. succumbing to frequent colds)
- Recurring bladder or vaginal infections
- Chronic tiredness
- Sensitivity to a food or foods
- Inflammatory diseases e.g. arthritis, gout
- Autoimmune diseases e.g. psoriasis, coeliac; Hashimoto's
- Asthma and allergies
- Metabolic syndrome (Syndrome X or pre-diabetes)
- Diabetes (type 1 or type 2)
- Obesity

If any of the above symptoms sound familiar or if they are getting to be a clingy friend that keeps paying regular visits, then perhaps it's time to look at what can cause these symptoms and take steps to show them the door! A leaky gut could well cause these problems. How this comes about continues to be the subject of many scientific studies. They show us how healing a leaky gut can stop the parade of niggles (and more dire consequences) in its tracks. Not surprisingly, the cure lies in a plant-based diet, improved stress control and maintaining a low-toxin environment.

Few people have any idea about what happens to their food once eaten. Most know that it will go down to the stomach and then through the bowels and out the other end. What actually happens is perhaps the most amazing journey that can be documented.

THE DIGESTIVE SUPER HIGHWAY

The digestive tract can be broken down into sections that the food must pass through, passing a tollgate after each stage of the journey:

Stage 1 goes from the mouth and down the oesophagus.
Stage 2 is the stomach
Stage 3 is the small intestine
Stage 4 is the colon (or large intestine) to the anus.

If digestion is a symphony, let's hope it's playing delightful Mozart rather than dissonant Schönberg! (Just for the record, I love both!) The orchestral players need to ensure they are following the composer's directions to get the intended result: time signature, key, tempo and pitch are vitally important. In our bodies the gallbladder, pancreas, thyroid gland and liver play similar important roles – secreting hormones and conducting the digestive process, thus ensuring that our bodies derive maximum benefit from the food we eat.

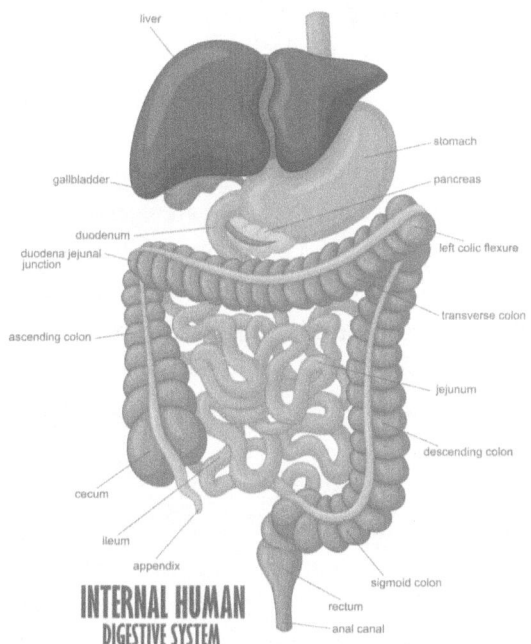

The Digestive System

We may not like to picture ourselves in the same way as the animals we watch devouring their prey on a David Attenborough wildlife documentary, but we have the same hardware as other predators: mouth with teeth and tongue and taste buds. Although I'd personally like to think humans have got a little more decorum than a lion wrenching flesh from a carcass, the fact remains that what happens at this first stage of the digestive journey in both cases is crucial to whether we get maximum nutrition and satisfaction from what we put in our mouths. Eating slowly isn't good just because it gives your body time to signal the brain to stop eating when full; it also creates prime conditions for optimum digestion. Essentially, poor digestion results in food passing through the digestive tract incompletely processed, which then allows it to play a starring role in the development of a leaky gut.

MICROBES AND TASTE

Taste is a phenomenon that arises from an intermingling of our senses. How a food smells is crucial to our perception of whether it tastes good or not. Then there's our tastebuds, but they aren't there just to help us enjoy our food – although that definitely happens. The five main taste types (sweet, bitter, umami, salty and sour) tell us what foods may or may not be safe for us to eat. Bitter foods, for example, have often proven to be poisonous, so this taste flags that a food may be potentially dangerous. Foods with a sweet taste indicate that they are energy rich. Oddly enough, taste receptors aren't only found on our tongue. There are taste receptors for sweet and bitter littered along the digestive super highway. The taste of a food helps deliver the message explaining exactly what the food is and what we can expect it to deliver in the way of macronutrients (carbohydrates, fats, proteins). The rest of the digestive system then prepares for the arrival of these particular foods.

Once a mouthful of food has slithered down the oesophagus and into the stomach it's time for the stomach acids and stomach muscle contractions to break it down. It is an amazing fact that each type of food comes with it's own user's manual. From the moment food enters your mouth it sends signals to the brain and the intestines instructing the body on exactly what it needs to process it. How long the food remains in the stomach and intestines forms part of these instructions.

AN INNER-GALACTIC WORLD – our science fiction-like interior

Unless we have eaten something problematic, we are not usually conscious of food once it leaves the stomach and enters the small intestine: out of sight, out of mind. Our parasympathetic nervous system (PSNS) takes over so we aren't consciously distracted by decisions involving what to do with all the stuff we've put in out mouths, but this is where things start to get truly interesting.

The small intestine is where most of the nutrition from our food is extracted and created. Yes, created – we don't get our nutrients just from what we eat. The food, or chyme as it is now called (pronounced *kyme*), is broken down by enzymes and bile acids into smaller, more absorbable components. At this stage molecules small enough to pass through the lining of the gut are formed. The gut lining is like a computer firewall, with sentinels that only allow molecules with the right visas to pass through into the bloodstream where they are used as nutrition. It is when chemical hackers penetrate the gut's firewall that things go awry, allowing a leaky gut to develop. Damage caused by a leaky gut can then impair our ability to manufacture nutrients essential to health and weight maintenance. Let's see how this happens....

The small intestine is very long. It varies from population to population, but in most people it is about 6 metres (20 feet) long! The structure of the small intestine is such that if you flattened and spread it out, it would have an area of about 250 square metres (850 square feet), which is about the size of a tennis court! It is this massive surface area that enables it to absorb nutrients. The surface of the small intestine is not just a smooth tube of muscle: it is covered with tiny projections called villi which are, in turn, covered by microvilli that look like tiny hairs. These features all play a role in the absorption of nutrients, but in the rough and tumble of this inner world they can easily be damaged. When they are in poor condition they contribute to leaky gut and some quite sinister diseases.

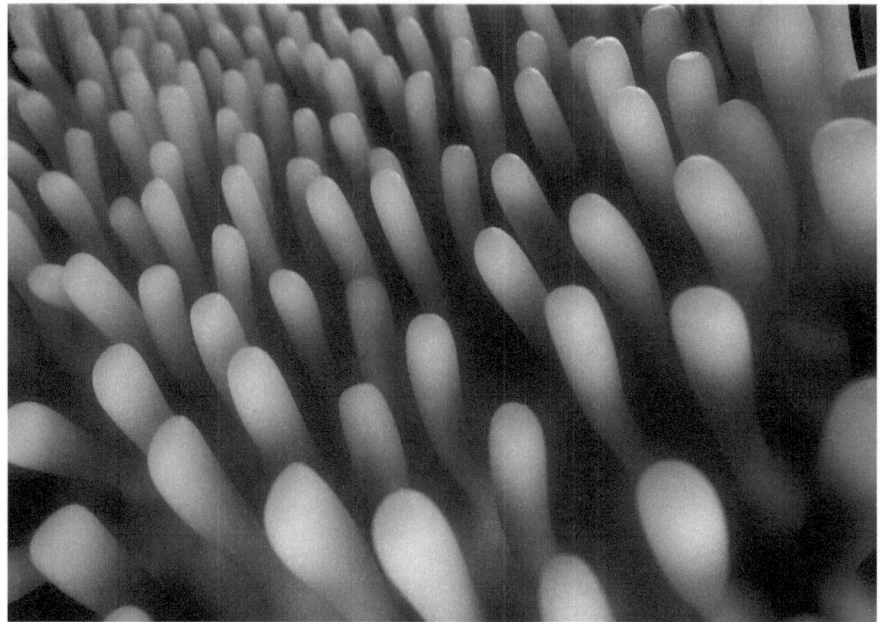

Villi of the intestinal wall

Each and every part of the digestive tract has its functions and all are important to our health. Hippocrates, who lived nearly 2,500 years ago, is claimed to have said, 'All disease begins in the gut'. Modern nutritional science seems to be bearing out his hypothesis.

What makes a gut healthy or otherwise? Short answer – the trillions of microbes that live there. Our insides are inhabited by microbes including, bacteria, fungi, protozoa and viruses. Collectively, they are known as the microbiome. If you've ever had a case of the runs, then you'll know that although most of these microbes are beneficial, some definitely are not. If you are overweight or have an autoimmune disease you probably have too many less-than-helpful microbes. The composition of your microbiome depends on your diet, the medicines you take, how stressed out you are and what toxins you have been exposed to. We'll cover these factors in more detail later on, but at this stage you need to understand that this is where the real action is at – your gut is the factory where your health or ill-health is forged.

The large intestine (the colon) is a much tidier affair than the small intestine. Its main functions are to reabsorb fluids and prepare waste for elimination from the body. It might surprise you that 40 per cent of everything that leaves your body is not food remnants, but gut bacteria and dead cells! Once we have excreted the waste the journey is over, but like the aftermath of a roller coaster ride, the consequences of the journey may be felt long after the ride has finished.

LET'S GET A TAKE AWAY....

1.

Much of what we were taught about nutrition since the 1950's has been shown to be wrong. Eating according to official guidelines has contributed to the obesity and autoimmune epidemics as well as to the increasing incidence of mental ill health.

2.

Eating according to official guidelines as represented by the food pyramid is not a recipe for good health. Quite the opposite, it can lead to Leaky Gut Syndrome and the diseases associated with that. Turning the pyramid on its head and 'eating upside down' can solve the problems associated with a leaky gut.

3.

Modern diseases, such as obesity, type 2 diabetes, autoimmune diseases and mental health disorders can usually be turned around, even cured, by repairing the gut and keeping it healthy.

4.

Poor dietary choices, trauma, stress, medications and antibiotic use can cause Leaky Gut Syndrome which promotes inflammation in the body and leads to a raft of modern day afflictions.

5.

The microbial gremlins in our guts play a crucial role in achieving and maintaining optimum physical and mental health. The more bad food choices we make, the more bad gremlins we will have. We may not notice their impact when we're younger but our bad choices can come home to roost in the form of disease at some point in our lives.

6.

The food we choose to eat determines how healthy our gut is. The health of our gut determines much of our overall health. Choose wisely.

CHAPTER 2

YOUR LEAKY GUT

There are three main culprits in the leaky gut scenario: poor diet, medications and stress, all of which knock the microbiome out of balance. However, as mentioned previously, our health problems actually start in the mouth and not just with the type of foods we choose. Not taking the time to chew properly is problematic for our guts and our subsequent health. This is one of my personal failings as I eat way too quickly. To many of us meals are a blur – something to be ticked off the list so we can move on to 'more important things'. Wrong.

DUNGEON DWELLERS:
the inhabitants in the depths of our intestines

The trillions of microbes that make up our gut flora are collectively known as the microbiome. They are an alien world within our world. In fact, of all the cells that make up the human organism, only about 10 per cent of them are actually human. The rest belong to the microbes we live with and which we couldn't live without.

We have been talked into fearing germs. Advertising for cleaning products, hand sanitisers, mouth wash and air fresheners feed on our fear of pathogens and becoming ill through contact with the unseen world of the microbe. These hideous micro criminals lie in wait, like a big cat ready to pounce and make us sick. It's true that some microbes will definitely make you ill and maybe even kill you. Famous culprits such as *Clostridium difficile (C. diff)*, salmonella and *E. Coli* can and do cause trouble. Many of these pathogens are part of the normal flora found in our bodies and when kept in check they cause no trouble at all. It is only when the balance between the beneficial and harmful microbes is upset that the picture changes.

Pathogens only make up a tiny fraction of the approximately 1,000 bacterial species that we are home to and we interact with thousands more in the environment. The vast majority of microbes in our world are not only beneficial but indispensible to our health and our lives in general. Anyone who has enjoyed yoghurt or cheese, beer, wine or sauerkraut can only be thankful for the actions of microbes.

Our micro inhabitants play vital roles in many of our basic bodily functions. Apart from their essential role in digestion, they also have profound effect on our weight, our level of pain and inflammation as well as our emotions and mental health.

There is a helpful, symbiotic relationship between humans and their gut microbes. Like accomplished interior designers these microbes furnish us with an enormous array of vitamins and other metabolites that keep us healthy and functioning. On the other hand it is we who provide them with the lounge room, kitchen and living space they require to thrive and multiply.

So what exactly do they do for us and how can we help them keep themselves and us in peak condition?

THE SEE-SAW OF LIFE – keeping a steady hand on the tiller

When the microbiome is in a balanced state, the integrity of the gut is maintained and we are generally in good health. In such a condition the microbes in the gut are predominantly of the beneficial kind and they keep the trouble-makers (pathogens) in check. The good guys thrive and there is little opportunity for the bad guys to bully the other kids in the playground and kick them out of the sand box. On the other hand, when the microbiome is unbalanced the tough kids or other miscreants kick a hole in the fence and go on a rampage, getting into places they have no right to be.

Like the secret service, the small intestine keeps a pre-emptive eye on microbial terror suspects and tries to stop them from crossing the border into our bloodstream, all without offending their rights and causing an international incident. It has to oversee the production of essential metabolites such as short-chain fatty acids and vitamins and usher them across the gut barrier into the bloodstream while at the same time preventing microbial terrorists from sneaking past security check points.

Unlike a medieval fortress with walls two metres thick to it help stand up to bombardment and potential breaches by the enemy, the gut wall itself consists of only a single layer of cells called the epithelium. It is vitally important that the integrity of this wall is maintained, but as we shall see, the invaders come well-armed and they won't hold off on dirty tricks either - some of our best known adversaries pull off Trojan horse capers with great finesse. This thin barrier of cells often caves into the onslaught of the North American or modern-day lifestyle. The friendlier contingents of our gut flora can be decimated in the battles we fight against the barrage of modern living. Such a diet leaves us open to the pathogens that make us sick.

BATTLE SCARS – Our microbiota and the immune system

The gut wall, or epithelium, is only one cell thick and covered in a layer of mucous. This may sound gross but it is this mucous layer that protects the gut wall and makes it harder for the pathogenic microbes to reach the bloodstream. The mucous layer is home to one of our BFF microbes called *Akkermansia muciniphila*. If your population of *Akkermansia muciniphila* is decimated along with your other good microbes, then your gut is in trouble, and so are you. This scenario can be brought on by something as simple as a course of antibiotics or steroids, trauma or long-term poor eating choices. Once the home turf of these friendly microbes has been left vacant, bad microbes seize the opportunity and take over the prime gut real estate. They now have access to the unprotected gut wall itself. The nasty microbes shout in jubilation when they see they are on the home stretch without an immune system soldier in sight.

The cells of the epithelium are normally so closely joined that only the tiniest of molecules can slip between them and cross over into the bloodstream. It is crucial that metabolites (small molecules like vitamins, enzymes and short-chain fatty acids) are able to do this, as the body's cells need them in order to function.

There are three main short-chain fatty acids (SCFAs): acetate, propionate and butyrate. They all play an important role in our overall health and especially the health of the gut itself. Butyrate is especially important for maintaining the integrity of the gut wall. It is like the fabled little Dutch boy who plugged a hole in the dyke with his finger: this SCFA repairs gaps that appear in the gut wall thus preventing larger and more dangerous molecules from crossing into the bloodstream where they can be carried throughout the body and cause all sorts of havoc and sometimes irreversible damage in the form of inflammation, chronic disease and mental ill-health.

People who have chronic diseases such as obesity, arthritis or any of the autoimmune diseases, usually have dysbiosis, which means that the balance between their good gut bacteria (Bacteroidetes) and their bad gut bacteria (Firmicutes) is out of kilter, with the harmful bacteria in much higher proportions than is healthy for us.

The bad gut bacteria have a chemical in their coats called lipopolysaccharide or LPS and it is LPS that plays a major role in making the gut leaky. So the more 'bad' bacteria there are in your gut, the leakier it will be. *If you eat a lot of animal fats then you increase the amount of LPS in your gut, which in turn activates the immune system causing the inflammation that lies behind the majority of modern day diseases.* Even if you are not vegan it is wise to limit the amount of animal fat in your diet if you want to control the bad bacteria in your gut and prevent and/or heal the diseases associated with leaky gut. There are plenty of other, healthy fats to enjoy as part of a well-balanced diet.

A BIG FAT LIE

At this point I need to point out that animal fat in itself is actually not bad for you. Back in the middle of last century saturated fat got a really bad rap and was blamed for causing heart disease. As a result millions of people changed to eating a diet very low in saturated fats and instead started consuming polyunsaturated fats such as sunflower and other seed oils. There will be more on this topic in Chapter 4. The obesity epidemic is clear evidence that the 'fat makes you fat' idea was not just deeply flawed, but actually harmful. Dr David Perlmutter, who is the author of several books on this topic, says that the dietary advice given by the USDA at that time has killed more people than World War I and World War II combined. Unfortunately, governments around the world followed the lead of the Americans and now the consequences are costing most Western nations many millions of dollars annually in health costs and lost productivity.

Based on the fact that humans survived for scores of millennia on oils from fruit, nuts and animals, it is safe to say that continuing in this vein is probably not going to hurt you unless you eat way too much of it. You could say: *if the oil is from fruits and nuts, eat it up, if it comes from seeds, then leave it be.*

THE IMMUNE SYSTEM IS NOTHING TO BE SNEEZED AT

But back to the gut which is home to about 60 per cent of our immune system. We are all familiar with the actions of the immune system: sneezing, rashes, asthma, itchy eyes, and so on. All these signs of an immune reaction are caused by the chemicals released when we come into contact with something we are allergic to. The master controller of allergies in the body is a chemical called Immunoglobulin E (IgE). People with allergies, chronic fatigue syndrome, candidiasis, asthma, eczema, autism and many other conditions have high levels of IgE that results in an overactive immune system and subsequent inflammation.

When you are allergic to something you can take an anti-histamine to make the symptoms disappear. It is unfortunate that pathogenic bacteria in the *Staphylococcus*, *E. coli* and *Proteus* families create too much histamine in the gut. This causes allergies, addiction, low blood pressure, sleep problems and hormonal changes. Having suffered from most of these maladies caused by a compromised immune system, I can tell you that not being able to breathe because of asthma and being hospitalised for low blood pressure are not insignificant problems. I can also tell you that many of my allergic problems, especially my asthma, are now generally a thing of the past. I no longer need a preventative medication based on steroids to control it, which is a good thing because steroids also cause significant harm to the gut lining.

Visible allergies make us aware that our bodies are fulfilling their protective role of keeping us safe from intruders. However, it is the allergies we can't see and their by-products that can cause us so much grief. Most of what we term age-related and lifestyle diseases are caused by the body's immune response to repeated breaches of the epithelium, whether that is by microbes that have kicked down the fence and gone off piste or by the incursion of products we are sensitive to, like wheat, dairy or medications. These things are a direct cause of Leaky Gut Syndrome and their presence results in chronic low-grade inflammation throughout the body.

Having a test for food allergies is crucial to detecting antagonists to the gut lining. Finding that I was allergic to wheat (not gluten!) and rye made all the difference in being able to overcome a weight loss plateau at 102kg (225 lb). I deleted them from my diet and off came another 30kg (66lb)!

CANDIDA – A tenacious and serious problem

There are other causes of leaky gut such as the microbe *Candida albicans*, a yeast that normally lives in our bodies without causing any problems. If we eat a diet high in carbohydrates, use antibiotics as well as some other medications, then this yeast can easily get out of control and cause significant harm to every part of the body, including the heart and the brain. Its actions are silent and insidious because apart from the occasions when it causes thrush or jock itch it usually lingers in cells throughout our bodies. It is pernicious because the damage it does is massive yet it is hard to recognise and hard to fix.

The worst thing about Candida is the fact that it is capable of putting down roots (called hydrae) directly into the gut wall. These roots are directly responsible for making holes in the epithelium, making it porous and allowing all sorts of unwanted substances to enter your bloodstream and negatively affect your health. If I had managed to finish the treatment for Candida back in the 1980's, many of my later health problems may not have arisen or at least been kept in check.

Taking a course of antibiotics will drastically affect most of the bacteria in our guts, wiping out some species for good and making it hard for others to repopulate. But *Candida albicans* is not a bacterium, so when the antibiotics have done their job and cleared out bacterial gut real estate, there is plenty of space left for the yeast to grow and thrive. This is why so many people have an outbreak of thrush, tinea or loose bowels after a course of antibiotics. A course of steroids or even using steroid-based medications such as those used for asthma will have much the same effect.

HEALING A LEAKY GUT – Hey, doctor, leave them pills alone!

Firstly, it's going to take time to heal. It can take a while, sometimes years, for a leaky gut to develop, and according to Dr Sandra Cabot of Cabot Health and Dr Natasha Campbell-McBride of the Cambridge Nutrition Clinic, it's going to take at least six to twelve months or more of dedicated dietary regulation to bring about some healing and turn the problem around. What you will also find is that the answer to your problems does not lie in taking a particular pill or supplement. Only diet and lifestyle can help. *There is no pharmaceutical that will heal your leaky gut* but there is one that you should astutely avoid unless you are going to be on death's doorstep without it: antibiotics.

One of the best things you can do to heal your gut and improve your health is to avoid antibiotics. Notice I said avoid, not exclude. Unfortunately, antibiotics are too frequently prescribed for maladies that do not require them at all. A while back I had what were quite obviously symptoms of an underactive thyroid (hair loss, cracked heals, dry skin, weight gain) and I was absolutely flabbergasted when the GP gave me a script for antibiotics – like that was going to help! In fact, when you read the section on hormones you will understand that the antibiotics could have made the problem worse. I got opinions from two other doctors and yes, it was hypothyroidism. Many people go the doctor with a cold and expect a script for antibiotics. Colds are caused by viruses, not bacteria, so taking the antibiotics won't help the cold at all. What they will do is destroy your gut bacteria and promote a leaky gut, cause weight gain, compromise your immune system, possibly give you a good dose of thrush and help you build antibiotic resistance. Sweet.

Because everything you put in your mouth must pass through your digestive tract, your diet can also be a severe source of antagonism to your gut and its resident bacteria. Most of the foods we eat today come from four main sources: modern wheat, modern meat, corn and GM soy, all of which can cause your gut to become permeable. Avoiding these foodstuffs will greatly enhance your prospects of healing the source of your obesity, your autoimmune disease, your age-related disease, your allergies or mental health issues.

WHAT'S GOOD FOR YOUR GUT?

Studies have shown that increasing the number of *Akkermansia muciniphila* bacteria in your gut will help enormously. These, and most of the other beneficial bacteria thrive on fibre, especially soluble fibre. For this reason you should increase the amount of fibre-rich foods in your diet. Such bacteria have a particular yen for asparagus, leeks, bananas and other foods that have soluble fibre (pretty much all vegetables), so they're not exactly hard to please. These microbes ferment the fibre and produce by-products including butyrate, which is one of those extremely beneficial short-chain-fatty-acids (SCFA). You may have heard of these before as they get quite a bit of press. This beautiful metabolite is counter-inflammatory in the gut and helps prevent obesity, colon cancer and autoimmune diseases. It does this by protecting the gut wall and making it less prone to becoming leaky. Along with vitamins K1 and K2 it also protects the lining of our veins and arteries.

Media campaigns based on the food pyramid have brainwashed most of us into thinking that grains are essential for fibre. In fact, the type of fibre found in grains, especially wheat, can be very harsh on the gut, making it sore and inflamed. The modern world is full of people who suffer painful diverticulitis, colitis and Irritable Bowel Syndrome. Is it any wonder?

Many studies have revealed that animal-based diets result in lower levels of SCFAs, so such diets provide less protection against the diseases we all want to avoid, like cancer, dementia and heart disease. This could be one reason why Westerners, with their high animal-content diets have greater rates of such diseases than populations whose diets are predominantly plant-based. Westerners have fewer microbes for processing complex carbohydrates, so we are simply not as efficient at processing them and we produce fewer beneficial SCFAs. There are some studies that show dairy, especially full-fat dairy, to be a source of the SCFA butyrate, but as you will discover, most of this benefit is eroded by its negative effects, such as a much-increased risk of many common cancers. Eating your vegies and ensuring you have sufficient vitamin B12 and vitamin D in your diet are still the best tactics for losing weight and maintaining optimal health.

WHEN IS A CALORIE NOT A CALORIE?

If the balance of microbes in your gut is weighted in favour of the bad guys, the Firmicutes, you are likely to have weight problems. Why? Because many of these bacteria demand we eat processed carbohydrates and when we do them the favour of providing their favourite, bread roll, pizza, pasta or beer they have the hide to be greedy little beggars by crunching calorie numbers differently from the good guys. They extract more energy from those foods than other microbes. The difference may only be small, but from little things big things grow: in a year you might only gain 2 or 3 kilos (6 to 10 lb), but over a few years this adds up to significant middle-aged spread – and you don't even have to be middle-aged!

GRAIN, GRAIN GO AWAY, COME AGAIN ANOTHER DAY –
why omitting grains helps heal your gut

In general, it is wise to avoid grains while you are trying to heal your gut. As I mentioned above, finding that I was allergic to wheat and rye and eliminating them from my diet made a world of difference to my weight loss efforts and to my health in general. For most people this will only be a temporary measure, but for many people, abstaining from them improves their health so much that they either quit them for good or only indulge on special occasions. Keep in mind that a food allergy is different from a food intolerance. With a food intolerance, a healed gut can usually tolerate such foods without any ill effect, especially if they are only eaten in small amounts and not too often.

GLUTEN

By avoiding grains you will also be avoiding a sneaky and omnipresent gut antagonist: gluten. Not many people are allergic to gluten – that is, they do not have coeliac disease, but many people, like me, have a sensitivity to gluten. Because it carries chemical labels that make it look similar to real enemies of the gut, the immune system becomes overly concerned about its presence and launches an inflammatory response. You may not get a full allergic reaction (almost instant catastrophic diarrhoea and gut pain), but it can overstimulate the immune system and you might get wind and bloating instead, sometimes only days later.

Exposure to gluten causes your body to increase the production of a protein called zonulin. Zonulin controls how tight the junctions are between the cells in your gut wall. Studies have shown that it could play a part in coeliac disease and type 1 diabetes. When we eat wheat, another protein called gliadin signals the body to produce more zonulin, which in turn causes the gut to become leakier, so it is important to avoid wheat and gluten-containing products (including personal care products) while trying to heal your gut. Read your labels!

In addition to the above, all grains come with a coating that causes significant distress to the gut: lectins. Lectins not only have a negative effect on your gut, but can also play havoc with your pancreas and thyroid. This is especially important to keep in mind if you have problems with your glucose metabolism (such as Syndrome X, pre-diabetes or type 2 diabetes). The thyroid helps control your rate of metabolism and if it is put out of whack you are likely to gain weight and have any number of side effects. Since eliminating wheat, rye and gluten products from my life, my thyroid has healed and I no longer need any medication - another major contributor to poor gut health bites the dust. Staying healthy is getting cheaper all the time!

DAIRY – not so healthy, not so innocent

And dairy? Well, it causes your body to produce mucous, which is a protective substance. This fact alone shows that the body is trying to protect itself from the irritation dairy products cause. As you would know from when you have had a cold, excess mucous can cause a significant amount of distress in the body. You will cough and sneeze to get rid of it. When the mucous lining in the gut gets too thick it makes it difficult for the vitamins produced by the bacteria to reach the gut wall and be absorbed. As a result you can develop nutrient deficiencies. A low GI vegan diet hinders the overproduction of mucous and improves the absorption of vitamins and other metabolites.

There is a lot of claim and counter claim surrounding dairy and calcium. While it is a good source of calcium, it is not the only source of calcium and there are many other plant sources that deliver as much, if not more, of this important mineral. Really, the choice is yours. If you follow a vegan lifestyle you will have no problems getting sufficient calcium and you will do your gut a favour in the process. Eating kale, for example, delivers the most calcium of any food as well as the side-nutrients required to deliver it to your system. In fact, you will notice that eating a vegan diet will cover all the crucial gut-healing bases. Removing grains from the diet, either temporarily or permanently, will also speed the recovery process.

CLEAN EATING

I ran into a former colleague in the supermarket one day and I told her how well she looked. She had just come through a round of chemotherapy and I was surprised that she was in good spirits and manifesting good health. She told me that her daughter had been staying with her and that they had been 'eating clean'. Now, this was new to me. She explained that it was avoiding foods that contained chemicals or which had been grown using genetic modification - kind of like a suped up organic diet. I decided that it was probably worth investigating, so I researched it.

When I discovered how toxic many food additives were and the effect of systemic herbicides and insecticides on the integrity of the gut, I decided it was time to eat clean, too.

I realised that even the most serious attempt at eating a clean diet was bound to be thwarted – it just isn't possible to avoid every chemical all the time. But I figured that omitting as many of these problematic substances from my diet, personal care products and household was worth the effort. Reducing the toxic load on the body reduces stress and improves gut health. That's what we want!

E NUMBERS – Is E for Evil? And is E171 a bona fide nasty?

We've all seen them – we pick up a pack of our favourite biscuits or yummy treat only to find a slew of E numbers appended to the list of ingredients. 'E' for Evacuate! 'E' for Evil? Actually 'E' is for Europe because the system was introduced by the European Food Safety Authority. Not all E numbers are nasty. E100 is turmeric and E160c is paprika, which are both natural. But some E numbers are believed to cause cancer and have been banned for human consumption. For instance, E123 (Amaranth), which gives foods a dark red colour, is banned in the USA and is only allowed in low concentrations in Australia and Europe. E102 Tartrazine is a yellow colouring (also mixed with blue dyes to create greens) that has been linked to asthma and other sensitivities.

Interestingly, a link was found between certain mixtures of E numbers and hyperactivity in children – we've all heard of children who go crazy after eating green jelly, for instance! Knowing what we do about the role of the gut in ADHD and other mental health disorders, one could wonder what effect these substances are having on the guts of these children.

Very recently a University of Sydney study found that E171 had a "substantial and harmful" influence on human health. E171 is Titanium Dioxide nanoparticles and you'd be right to zero in on the nanoparticle epithet. Whenever 'nano' is prefixed to a word it means super-duper teeny-weeny in size. Nanoparticles are so small they can unobtrusively move from the gut, through the gut wall and into the bloodstream. If you have a leaky gut this can be especially problematic. The University of Sydney study showed that E171 impacts the gut microbiota with negative outcomes. It doesn't change the composition of gut microbiota like antibiotics, but it does alter their activity which leads them to form a biofilm (bacteria that are stuck together). Biofilm has been shown to be a contributing factor in inflammatory bowel diseases and bowel cancer. In fact, numerous studies have highlighted the role of nanoparticles in diseases ranging from cancer to eczema, asthma, and autoimmune diseases. The effects of E171 have prompted the French government to ban its use from late in 2019. Message here? Steer clear of it if you can!

VITAL NOURISHMENT FROM THE GUT

Our gut bacteria produce some very important nutrients. The water-soluble B vitamins including B1, B2, B3, B5, B6, B12, folate and biotin are essential to help convert carbohydrates to glucose and make energy. If your microbiome is out of whack and producing insufficient B vitamins then you may well feel lethargic, lack energy or have unrefreshing sleep. The link between B vitamins and energy production in the body cannot be dismissed. In a 15-year trial, researchers at Gothenburg University in Sweden showed that injections of the biologically active form of B12 (methylcobalamin) can be helpful in alleviating the debilitating effects of Chronic Fatigue Syndrome (CFS).

In fact, our entire nervous system is reliant on the B vitamins to function properly. This is why they play a role in keeping diseases like MS and Parkinson's at bay; B12 in particular because it is intimately involved with providing the protective cover of each and every nerve cell (the myelin sheath). B vitamins are also essential in the development of red blood cells that transport oxygen around the body, and B5 helps make the hormones that help control most of our bodily functions such as metabolism and reproduction. Even more crucially, niacin and B12 play a role in making new DNA, and folate is a major player in epigenetics – where the environment, including stress and nutrition, are able to regulate your genes, turning them on and off in a process called methylation. More about this in Chapter 5.

Gut bacteria are also directly responsible for producing the K vitamins. Like most things in this world we should strive for balance. Vitamin K1 is a good example of this. Without it our blood will not clot, but too much of it will cause the blood to be thick and possibly block blood vessels, which can be catastrophic. Vitamin K2 on the other hand, has a very special role to play. More and more research highlights its role in disease, and its importance in keeping us healthy has become ever more apparent. Some authorities claim it is the 'missing link between diet and several killer diseases'. K2 partnered in a dance with vitamin D, plays a role in determining whether the calcium in our bodies ends up in our bones and teeth or in our tissues and blood vessels where it can lead to plaque formation and blockages. If our levels of K2 are optimum, the calcium predominantly heads for our skeleton and we avoid hardening of the arteries (atherosclerosis). It may also lower the risk of osteoporosis and improve dental health.

As you can see, these vitamins are vital to our wellbeing and the gut is the factory - our bacteria make them for us. It pays to treat our gut microbes well.

And what about vitamin D? Well, to start with, it's not actually a vitamin at all – it's a hormone – but when it was first discovered the scientists thought it was a vitamin and the tag stuck. Most people know that we get vitamin D predominantly from sunlight. Nowadays people spend more and more time indoors and even professional athletes such as surfers, who spend a lot of time in the sun, can still become vitamin D deficient because they use sunscreen. Vitamin D can also be sourced from eggs, fatty fish like salmon, beef liver, some dairy products and oddly enough orange juice, soy milk and cereals.

Keeping Vitamin D at optimum levels has been shown to have a positive effect on metabolic syndrome. If you are low in vitamin D you are doing your microbiome no favours. JJ Oppenheim and his colleagues at the National Cancer Institute in Maryland have shown that vitamin D lowers the production of defensins in the mucous lining of the gut wall, which is a good thing because defensins are anti-microbial. Of course, they have their benefits, and play a role in our health, but as usual the positives only last as long as the balance is kept. Too high a level of defensins ups the action of the immune system, which inevitably increases inflammation and the diseases related to it.

Vitamin D is also crucial to sustaining processes that affect our mental health. Keeping levels optimal will assist in stabilising mental function. Avoiding roller coaster-like highs and lows in mood is crucial to our long-term mental health and helps maintain better relationships at home, at work and at play.

We live in an unnatural world and like most people I spent a lot of time indoors and avoided the direct sun when out. As a consequence I was severely deficient in vitamin D. I started to take a supplement in drop form, which fixed the problem. More recently I have started eating my lunch outdoors and I no longer need the supplements, except in the summer when it is just too hot in Australia to venture out.

WHAT'S OUR TAKE AWAY?

1.
An unhealthy gut is a leaky gut. A leaky gut is the root cause of most modern ailments including obesity, autoimmune diseases and mental ill health.

2.

There are no pills you can take to heal a leaky gut. Only diet and lifestyle choices can do that.

3.

The gut is home to 60 per cent of our immune system. Our guts need to be in good shape to help prevent allergies and autoimmune diseases and to keep us in peak mental health.

4.

Microbes make up 90 per cent of the human body. Some are dangerous pathogens that make us sick but most are beneficial and even essential to our existence. We need to look after our microbes.

5.

The types and balance of microbes in the gut determine how many calories we absorb from our food and therefore our weight. Eating unprocessed plant foods ensures that there is a higher proportion of "good" to "bad" microbes in the gut, thereby helping the body to lose weight.

6.

Dairy and grains cause significant damage to the gut and are best avoided.

7.

Clean eating can lower the toxic load on the gut and give it a better chance to heal.

8. Know your E numbers and steer clear of the trouble makers.

9.

Eating foods high in soluble fibre is essential for gut health. Foods like asparagus and bananas ferment in the gut and feed the helpful bacteria that produce short chain fatty acids. SCFAs help repair damage to the gut lining and maintain its integrity.

10.

Gut microbes produce vitamins, neurotransmitters and other metabolites essential to our wellbeing. These metabolites play a critical role in how we think about food and how we metabolise it. The gut needs plenty of vegetable fibre to supply the necessary substances to sustain health.

CHAPTER 3

YOUR WEIGHT

Obesity. Well, we all know what makes you fat, and it's all your own fault:

- You eat too much – too many calories
- You eat too many fatty, rich foods
- You don't exercise enough
- You're lazy

You have to use more calories than you eat. Right? Calories in. Calories out.

Let's just hold the order on that serving of smug condemnation with the extra dollop of self-righteousness, shall we….

Of course, all of these things in certain combinations can be part of the problem, but let's look at the following list and compare:

- Your combination of gut microbes helps you absorb more calories than a lean person's

- Your gut microbes affect your mental health and give you extra barriers to hurdle such as depression and an inclination to eat poor food combinations
- Your gut microbes cause you to crave the foods *they* thrive on
- Your genes, epigenetics and your personal history of stress and trauma predispose you to put on weight
- Your genes predispose you to have an aversion to exercise

Spot the difference? That's right. Fat people saying that they don't understand why they put on weight just by looking at food is not just an attempt to shift the onus of responsibility from themselves to some fat fairy. I can't count how many times some total stranger has called out my supposed self-serving weakness and gluttony in public by making fun of my fat! Like they have a monopoly on righteous self-restraint and an inside view to my metabolic world!!

An astounding amount of research over the last few years confirms that fat people aren't always just making it up – they really do not understand the reason for their excess weight. For that matter, neither do those rude so-and-sos that call them out on it either!

More and more carefully controlled studies using ever better research technology show that obesity is not as simple as calories in versus calories out. If it were, then all those people who exercise their hearts out and stick to their doctor's diets wouldn't struggle to lose weight and, morale-destroyingly, gain it back once lost. If exercise as a method of weight loss worked then those overweight people who do an hour or more of exercise every day and watch their diets should be in good shape. Tim Spector, author of the hugely influential book called *The Diet Myth* succinctly states: 'trying to lose weight by exercise alone is futile'. Just as importantly, in her book *10% Human* Alanna Collen reminds us that, 'Counting "calories in" is not as simple as keeping track of what a person eats. More accurately, it is the energy content of what the person *absorbs*.' So how does this all work, and what does it mean for those of us who wage a perpetual battle against the scales?

CALORIES IN – CALORIES OUT, DOESN'T ADD UP

Firstly, if you want to lose weight, it is logical to assume that you have to use more calories than you consume. To a certain extent that is true, however, this logic is based on Newtonian-aged thinking where every action had an equal and opposite reaction. It is completely understandable; just do the sums. The trouble is that the Newtonian age was the age of the industrial revolution, where machines and their inventors were demigods. Human beings are not machines. No matter how many times we hear things like 'digestive system' or analogies between the brain and a computer, science shows us that we are much more complicated than the most complex of machines: we are quantum beings.

The upshot of this concept is that we may be trying to measure one thing, but we cannot understand or take into account effects of processes that we have little knowledge of, many of which we have never even contemplated the existence of. Our knowledge is in no way complete. Think of the times when scientists have thought that they have the answer to a problem and have implemented a strategy to counteract it, only to cause unforseen complications. The introduction of the cane toad into Australia is one fine example. Yes, the cane toads ate the cane beetles they were imported to dine on, but the consequences have been dire for our native species. Populations of some species are now endangered because they ended up on the cane toad's expanded menu.

What we can do, however, is take a good look at what the latest research tells us. Amazingly enough, it says that the answers we seek are actually in the past, from the time before humans tried to play God by creating foods and chemicals to fulfil every human desire and get around the problem that the human population was outgrowing its supply base. Time and again we are admonished by recent research to return to a time when our environment was natural, unadulterated and clean.

Many will want to argue about when this ideal pre-modern time ended – it all depends on which camp you're in, but for the purposes of this book I am going to contend that eating natural, unprocessed foods ceased to be a regular, normal thing about the time margarine was invented in 1869. Up until then, processed foods were uncommon and the most common food processing technique apart from cooking was the milling of grain. (Aptly enough, it was the classes that could afford the most highly processed grain that succumbed to what we would now call modern diseases, such as obesity). Even tinning food was a fairly new process at this stage and Coca Cola came onto the market only 23 years after margarine. It is worth stressing that these 'foods' are not natural – they are invented. In a strange twist of fate (or an insidious sleight of commercial hand) soda drinks would eventually come to cost less than the water used in their processing. Nothing natural was good enough anymore – man could improve on nature. Or was this just another case of a cane toad in sheep's clothing?

Some areas of the world are renowned for not succumbing to the wonders of modern living until quite recently; such places as Sardinia in Italy, Okinawa in rural Japan, Icaria in Greece and Nicoya in Central America, places we now call the Blue Zone, which are renowned as the homelands of the world's longest lived and healthiest people. What do all of these places have in common? These zones provide a relatively clean, rural, environment, the people who live there are semi-vegetarian, commonly eat legumes on a regular basis, have lifestyles that involve regular physical activity and their daily lives revolve around their family and community. These people consume fewer processed foods and use fewer chemicals in their lives.

I hear some readers saying, "I'm here for a good time, not a long time!" Fine, but the point of eating well and looking after your health is to preserve the life in your years not extend the years of your life.

The lifestyle of a contemporary urbanite is polluted to the hilt with chemicals in the air, the water, the food we eat, the clothes we wear and the attitudes we have about ourselves and others. Not surprisingly our homes tend to be cluttered and unhealthy. There are television shows that showcase the decline into consumerism hell, revealing lives that are packed to the rafters with unseemly amounts of consumer products and the emotional attachments that go with them. Even the air in our homes has to be 'freshened' with sprays and scents and candles (mainly toxic phthalates) that turn into formaldehyde and other lethal chemicals when they come into contact with the air they are meant to freshen and purify. Advertisements and capitalist cunning convince us that we need everything that modern industry can provide. Is it any wonder that our minds and bodies are rebelling?

Rebelling you ask? Yes. Obesity is a result of bodies that are stressed from being out of balance and they are taking a stand against the onslaught of chemical wizardry. Modern day disease epidemics are a sign that our bodies are waging losing battles. They are out of synch with the natural cycles and requirements of nature. Nature is not something separate from us. We are in it and it is in us. We are an integral part of it. Inseparable. It's when we try to separate and leverage ourselves out of the natural order than strife ensues.

I'm as guilty of consumerism as most other people. It's nice to have a gadget to do this or that – to supposedly make life easier. But does it really? If you've got to maintain it, clean it and store it, it had better be worth the money spent on it. Otherwise it is just more clutter that blunts the energy you have to live your life. I recently did a big clean out and had a garage sale to let go of un-needed items. Reducing the load on mind and body is a key way to achieving better health. Let me tell you, I feel lighter in spirit as well as in body now!

A very large part of the obesity epidemic arises because we have stopped eating natural, predominantly plant-based diets and have ventured off onto the road paved in gold by the capitalist trickster companies that are often referred to as 'big-pharma' and 'big food' with their glossy and cleverly conceived marketing tactics. Consideration for the welfare of the consumer is overshadowed by their end game: a fat bottom line. There are, of course, watchdogs and ombudsmen to mitigate the negative effects that such companies wreak on the unwary consumer, but these are only a Band-Aid on the blight of unscrupulous manufacturers and purveyors of products that are starting to destroy the very consumer base they claim to service. Nina Teicholz in her dogma-shattering book "The Big Fat Surprise" took the fight to the unscrupulous purveyors of all that is slowly killing us. Such companies push everything that is cheap, nasty, and easily produced to sate the desires of a planet-blighting human population.

ALL IS NOT LOST

The good news is that we now have scientific techniques that enable us to discern the causes of the misery that is obesity. Though in no way complete, our knowledge in this area is growing and it seems that the current crop of nutrition scientists have learnt a thing or two from their predecessors about fudging trial results to please corporate sponsors. In this digital day and age it's getting harder to camouflage such deception. Watchdogs and bloggers are being ever more vigilant and are exposing nefarious practices that harm the average consumer.

Modern research techniques are providing some answers to problems that previous dodgy science errantly supported. Continuing unabated, lobby groups and others with political and financial gain in mind are acting like spoiled brats who badger their parents at every turn and throw tantrums to blackmail them into allowing actions that really aren't in the best interests of anyone but themselves. There is no guarantee that the hoaxes perpetrated on the public at large over the last fifty years could not happen again, but hopefully we have learned from the past. It is also encouraging that researchers tell us to return to eating styles of a bygone era – eating styles that clearly brought mankind through prehistory and into the modern age and which can continue to sustain us without the inclusion of freakish man-made food-like substances. *The obesity epidemic is just as much a political and commercial issue as it is a personal one.*

So let's turn our attention to the points outlined at the start of this chapter. You will remember seeing the phrase 'gut microbes' on a couple of occasions. As it turns out, these microscopic creatures are essential to our existence and play a crucial role in how we fare on planet Earth.

10% HUMAN

It is estimated that only ten per cent of the cells in our bodies are human – the rest are microbes: bacteria, yeasts, fungi and so on. That's a bit of a turn up for the books! These microbes can be both beneficial and nasty. The nasty ones, pathogens, can even kill us if they get out of control. The good ones look after us and we can't live without them. Collectively, the microbes in our gut are called the microbiome.

Diet theories that do not take the microbiome into account are doomed to failure. Each person has their own unique set and balance of microbes. We are all different. This implies that a diet should be tailored to the individual, and in the future this may well be the way we learn to match our lifestyle to our needs. High fat diets or high carb diets or paleo diets might be good for one person, but not another. Certain diets may even be dangerous for specific individuals; a diabetic who continues to eat a diet high in processed carbohydrates like bread and pasta, wholegrain or not, is pouring oil on the fire of metabolic dysregulation. There are, however, some major ideas that apply to pretty much everybody.

As we have already seen, when it comes to microbes and weight loss and weight gain there are two types of bacteria we need to consider: Bacteroidetes and Firmicutes. The more bacteroidetes-type microbes you have the more likely you are to be lean and have fewer weight problems. Firmicutes, on the other hand, may have 'cute' in their name, but they are anything but. Yes, they have their role to play, and it is important that we have them, but once again it comes down to a question of balance and keeping these tricky little mobsters in their place. Bad food choices such as eating processed foods, vegan or not, will allow the bad guys to take over your gut territory and cause you health problems. *Please do not confuse veganism with healthy eating. You can be vegan and still eat a diet that contains a lot of processed foods, and that just isn't good for you. A low GI vegan diet on the other hand, that is based on eating wholesome, clean plant foods can lead to optimal health and deliver you from physical and mental ill health.*

Assistant Professor Peter Turnbaugh at the University of California, San Francisco, specialises in identifying the role of gut microbes in pharmacology and nutrition. He bred germ-free mice that had no microbiome of their own. He then transferred the microbes of obese mice into one group of the germ-free mice and microbes from lean mice into another group. Even though each group ate exactly the same type and amount of food, the two groups had outcomes that were poles apart. Those given microbes from the obese mice became obese and the others did not. This experiment showed that it was indeed gut microbes that had made the obese mice fat. Further studies showed that gut microbes determined how many calories and other nutrients the body absorbed from the food eaten. It was not so much calories in versus calories out, but how much energy was *absorbed* by the body. So this helps explain why two comparably-sized people of the same sex, eating the same diet and doing the same exercise can have dramatically different outcomes when it comes to maintaining their weight. So, to my friends out there who wondered how I could eat the same as them and do the same exercise with a totally different outcome, here is the answer to that part of the metabolic puzzle!

But this is not the whole story – not by a long way. Humans are magnificently complicated creatures and although this fledgling science has unearthed a myriad of new and intriguing concepts it is important to realise that the surface has only been scratched. It seems to be a truism that the more you know, the more you realise how little you actually know. Each new discovery throws up a new set of questions. So now, although it is clear that the microbiome definitely plays a role in weight gain, the question on researchers' lips is, 'why'?

GENETICS

Genetics is the science *du jour*. It excites the imagination of scientists, journalists and the public alike. Barely a day goes by when we don't hear or see a report about some important new discovery in this field. What really excites the scientific world though is the more recently developed science of epigenetics. This new science works at identifying how external factors such as the environment and psychology affect the genome – how trauma and diet, for example, can cause the genes to be turned on or off. There will be a much more in depth discussion on this topic later in the book, but right now it is interesting to note that it has been shown that a diet high in carbohydrates, especially early in life, can switch on the genes for fat storage and lead to obesity in later life. Think twice before giving your child those processed snacks like sodas, fruit juices, sandwiches and muesli bars! It could be setting them up for a life of obesity hell.

LEPTIN RESISTANCE

Another factor in weight gain is leptin resistance. Leptin is a hormone made by fat (adipose) cells and it is one of the factors that lets us know when we have had enough to eat. All things going well, we eat our food, our leptin levels rise and the brain recognises when we have consumed enough energy and says 'Stop, that's enough!' When things aren't functioning so well, leptin dons an invisibility cloak making it impossible for the brain to detect it. The brain can't 'see' the leptin and therefore thinks that we are in starvation mode. It then signals the body to increase insulin which sets in motion a cycle that helps the body store and lay down fat.

When your body thinks it's starving it begs you to feed it, so your appetite increases and you end up eating more. That's one reason why so many diets are hard to keep up and why so many people just cannot stick to a diet for the long haul. Your will power won't be enough when trying to fight your biology. That's why you need an eating regime that pretty much allows you to eat till you feel full; a diet that comprises mostly vegetables and a satisfying amount of good fats. Such an eating style goes a long way to fulfilling this need. That's one reason why a low-GI vegan regime worked for me.

LPS – Lipopolysaccharide WHAT A MOUTH FULL!

The fat cells in obese people are flooded with immune cells called phagocytes [pronounced *fajo-sites*]. These cells eat up invading cells that have alarmed the immune system. *For all intents and purposes this immune response means your fat cells are fighting an infection. Infection and inflammation go hand-in-hand and inflammation is at the heart of so very many diseases,* from diabetes to autoimmune diseases to heart disease: inflammation is the root cause. What can cause such pervasive chronic inflammation?

As you have already seen, a leaky gut is one major cause of inflammation that engulfs the body on a grand scale leading to disease. Professor Patrice

Cani of Imperial College in London delved into how this inflammation comes about. He found that gut microbes in obese people gave rise to the inflammation they experienced.

The demon in this story is LPS: lipopolysaccharide, which acts like a toxin when it gets into the bloodstream. Obese people tend to have high levels of this molecule in their blood. So where does it come from?

Various pathogenic (bad) gut bacteria like *E. coli*, *Shigella flexneri* and *Salmonella enterica* are coated with LPS to make their cell walls stronger and protect them from attack. This coating makes them hard to kill so they are potentially dangerous to our health. LPS elicits a very strong immune response if it crosses through a leaky gut into the bloodstream. This immune response is the inflammation that can devastate our bodies in the guise of any number of diseases. LPS also causes our bodies to store energy rather than burn it. In other words, it helps us put on weight.

Studies have shown that a diet very high in fat (especially polyunsaturates) promotes LPS, causing the gut to be leakier and leading to subclinical inflammation. However, as the man in the ad said, 'oils ain't oils' and although he was talking about car oil the principle holds true for edible oils as well. Australian author David Gillespie in his well-researched book 'Toxic Oils' gave very easy-to-follow advice: if the oil is from an animal, a fruit or a nut, then its good for you. If it's from a seed or some other source leave it on the shelf. *Margarine, Sunflower oil and 'vegetable' oils made from grains and seeds are all really bad for your health, especially when heated. These oils should NOT be used for cooking or baking.*

So what can prevent LPS from doing its damage? Our old friend the bacterium *Akkermansia muciniphila* will come riding to the rescue if you feed it its favourite foods such as asparagus, bananas and vegetables from the onion family. If this bacterium thrives in your gut it can help protect the epithelium, making it hard for the LPS-bearing bacteria to do their dirty work. An extra advantage of encouraging *Akkermansia* in your gut is that it helps make you more sensitive to the appetite-regulating hormone leptin. Bonus!

CONSTANT CRAVING

As we just saw, *Akkermansia* thrives on certain foods. All bacteria have their favourite take-away foods. In fact, our microscopic cellmates can even be the basis for our cravings. These sneaky little beggars demand their fill and get what they want by various means. They will even manipulate our psychology to do so. According to Joe Alcock from the University of New Mexico, microbes can 'hijack the dopamine-driven reward system' that makes us want more of a pleasurable thing whether that is sex, a muffin or heroin.

It turns out that we are like puppets on a string and our gut bugs are the puppet masters: they make us dance to their tune. They may even make us feel a little depressed or down until we eat the food *they* want. Once eaten we start to feel great again until the effect wears off and we have to eat more bread, bagel, crackers or whatever it is that they thrive on. This type of eating (which has been labelled 'hedonic eating') is also bad for our gut lining, making it leakier by activating the stress response. Stress results in steroid hormones such as cortisol entering the bloodstream and they can cause the gut lining to lose its integrity.

Cravings are also generated by eating certain foods. Grains that contain gluten and casein-containing dairy products release substances into our blood. These substances act on our brains as if we had used heroin or any other addictive drug. Look at the endings of their names and you will immediately be able to identify them for what they are: gluteomorphins and casomorphins. Just like morphine they trigger the brain's opioid receptors and as you can imagine, they have a powerful effect on our reward system. The more we consume of these foods the better we feel, despite any negative consequences that arise from their consumption such as obesity and flatulence. Any addict will tell you that it doesn't matter what your logical mind tells you, it's all about getting more of the drug. And so it is with these foods.

Back in the 1980's I used to joke that I was addicted to bread. I always knew that I craved it. Since the dietary guidelines told me that it was really good for me, especially if I ate the whole grain kind, I couldn't see anything wrong with it. Little did I suspect that I was feeding the nastier microbes in my gut and giving them permission to control me. This style of eating knocked around my metabolism and brought me closer to the metabolic cliff edge: for every two slices of bread I ate I was consuming the equivalent sugar value of a can of coke. Whoops! Thanks a lot gluteomorphins!

Casomorphins are found in dairy products. People who say they could never go vegan often cite cheese as the reason. 'I could never give up cheese', they say. The tug of love is strong, especially if you put the two morphine-like substances together in one meal. It's not a coincidence that macaroni and cheese along with pizza are two of the most popular dishes in the world. A double helping of morphine anyone?

It is well known that foods high in both fat and highly processed carbs such as pizzas, burgers and creamy pastas, can lead to food addiction. In ancient days our ancestors sought out foods that were high in fat, because fat can easily be used and stored by the body. And sweet foods like fruit and honey were either seasonal or difficult to acquire. Sweet meant energy-laden and if you ate enough carbohydrate it would be converted into fat reserves to help get you through lean times. Back then, who knew where the next meal was coming from? There were no supermarkets or convenience stores where you could duck in and pick up a high-fat, high-sugar treat at any time of day or night: not like now. As a result, we have an inbuilt predilection for high-fat, high-sugar combos. Great in times of severe deprivation. Not so great in the modern Western world.

In 2013 *Scientific American* magazine published an article entitled 'The Food Addiction' by Paul J Kenny. In it Kenny notes that endorphin blockers - drugs designed to alleviate addiction in drug-addicted individuals - can be used to alleviate food addiction too. This shows that food addiction, especially to processed foods containing wheat and dairy, is real. We are handcuffed to the same reward system as addicts of any other substance.

One of my clients, an offender whose crime was related to alcohol abuse, was intrigued by book notes on my desk and asked if he could have a copy. Later that day after he had read them, he came back to me and said; "Now

I know why I'm an alcoholic, why I crave beer, and how I can fix it." He was elated. He was hopeful he could now address his drinking problem, not just with the usual 12 steps, but by taking one extra step – changing his diet and healing his gut. One extra, 13th step. Hopefully it was a lucky one for him! He hasn't been back.

HABITS

Our bodies can crave processed foods with a high GI (glycaemic index) because of the reasons outlined above. The other problem might be that we become habituated to these foods. I was brought up on cheese and vegemite sandwiches for lunch or for a quick snack. A perfect storm for a future food addict: gluteomorphins in the bread, casomorphins in the cheese and yeast to feed *Candida albicans* (another habitual weight-gain offender) in the vegemite.

Even though I avoid these foods, I still occasionally want to let myself have them. I can daydream about the softness of the bread, the tang of the cheese and the salty umami of the vegemite and feel the sensation of gustatory satisfaction flood over me just by thinking about it. Old habits die hard. Just like a cigarette smoker will see himself putting a cigarette to his lips in his mind's eye, lighting it and dragging on it – something he imagines many times a day in the early stages of abstinence, I too will imagine biting into a soft, fresh cheese and vegemite sandwich. It's a conditioned response and hard to shake off. It makes you wonder who's really in control, you, your habits or those pesky little microbes in your gut.

Interestingly enough, changing your diet may seem like an extreme challenge, but by doing so, you will also change the types of bacteria in your gut and the proportions of good to bad bacteria improve. This will make some of the things that seemed so insurmountable before the change much easier to deal with. Sure you will miss certain things, but the mental anguish won't be as hard to overcome when you have the right microbes fighting on your side. The first few days might be hard and you will need will power, but it gets easier and easier as you take control instead of your microbes.

MACRO MANIACS : Carbs, fats and proteins

Low carb? High-carb? Low fat? High fat? What a conundrum. What's best? Well for some people, especially those who need to gain weight, high carb is not so bad. However, one thing has been definitively shown to be true: we all need to have a reasonable amount of good fats in our diet. The idea that saturated fat makes you fat is a dogma that has been proven to be entirely false. The claim was based on shonky research and perpetuated by misguided (and sometimes misled) authorities and the food industry.

What you will notice in any debate of this kind is that the terms 'high/low carb' or 'high/low fat' are bandied around like pucks in an ice hockey match. Most people understand high carb as being a diet weighted in favour of foods like potatoes, corn, grain products such as bread, pasta, crackers, pizza, pancakes, chips – basically all of our favourite and convenient foods. Strictly speaking however, carbs come under many more beneficial guises, such as apples, pears, oranges, bananas, grapes and the majority of other fruits as well as vegetables including sweet potato, pumpkin, carrot, cauliflower, onion, peas, lentils and so on. Most government health guidelines split the idea of carbohydrates into three more familiar categories: grains and grain products, vegetables and fruits. The current pyramid looks like this:

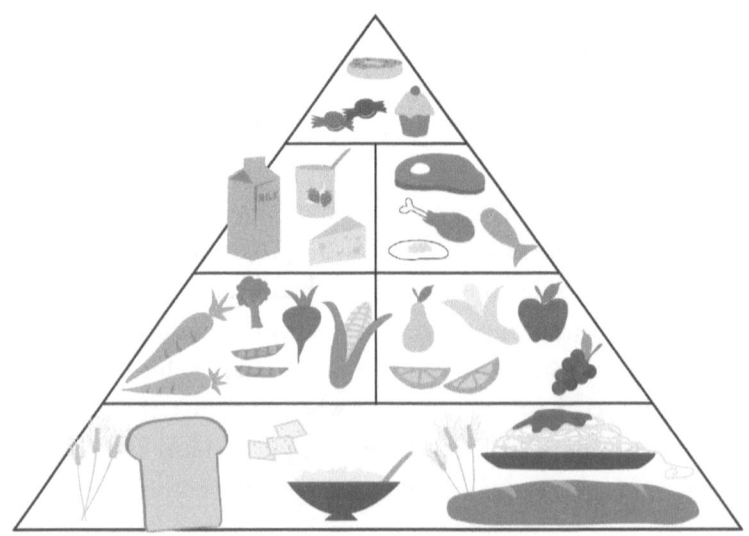

Current Food Pyramid

So, in their minds, the general population registers 'carbs' as different from fruits and vegetables.

If you adhere to the stricter and more encompassing definition: that fruit and vegetables are all part of the carbohydrate stratum in the food pyramid, then a high carb diet is indeed a prescription for health. The authors of 'The China Study', T. Colin Campbell and Tom Campbell argue that a diet of 80 per cent carbohydrates is optimal, and I agree. However, if this recommendation is quoted in isolation, as such things often are, it is less clear that the carbs should be mainly vegetables and fruit rather than processed foods, bread, potatoes, pasta, sweets and so on, which is what the majority of people see as carbs.

Most people would jump for joy on reading a recommendation of 80 per cent carbohydrate because they would see that as allowing them to persist in eating the standard Western diet they are accustomed to and which is slowly but surely killing them. Having said this, I believe that the prescription for health in The China Study, (based on the broader definition of carbs), is optimal for every human being and the planet. Eating by those guidelines would make most people vegan or near vegan. The authors call their diet WFPB (Whole Food Plant Based). I only discovered their definition many years after dubbing my diet Low GI Vegan. There are many similarities between the two, but differ mostly in respect to oils. I recommend a thorough reading of "The China Study". It could change your mind on many issues regarding nutrition and health.

Another major issue in the world of nutrition is fats. Fat is absolutely indispensible for our health. Each and every cell of our body needs fat and cholesterol to construct the cell membranes that keep us together and prevent us from becoming a pool of slime on the floor. To eliminate saturated fats and eat only mono and polyunsaturated fats in skimpy amounts as recommended by the food pyramid is to ask for trouble. The low fat campaign compelled populations throughout the Western world to drive down their intake of saturated fats in favour of margarines and polyunsaturated oils which easily convert to trans fats, which we now know are toxic and even lethal for us. We are told they are ideal for cooking, but they have low smoke points and easily turn into toxic trans fats. They are the worst oils you could possibly use for cooking, especially frying. The consequences are beginning to show themselves as increased incidences of diseases like Alzheimer's, MS and Parkinson's.

An interesting note is that if you want to change the ratio of Firmicutes to Bacteroidetes (fat versus lean) microbes in your gut, then try a diet low in processed carbs rather than a low fat diet. On a low-processed carb diet you don't have to lose as much weight before the changes to your gut take place. And a low fat diet makes it harder for positive changes to be made in your gut microbiome. Having saturated fat in your diet helps the gut lining to heal and become less permeable, especially if you reduce the amount of damaging grains and other foods that you may be sensitive to. All this will help solve weight problems, too. Although most saturated fats are of animal origin there are also plant sources such as coconut and nuts.

A BOUT OF INSANITY - Carbs versus the high-protein fad

In the blue corner: protein and in the red corner: carbs. Ever been to a fight where both opponents were laid flat on the canvas – a simultaneous knock out? Nup? Well, here it is. There are no winners here, so both sides had better just shake hands and man up to the fact that they both have an important role to play in nutrition and that they had better get on with a third sparring partner while they're at it: fats.

While devotees are at pains to support each of their boys, people around the world are getting ill and dying. It's not about which macronutrient is the best or most important, it's about working together so that everything is in balance and runs smoothly. Lose the gloves, the ropes and the self-important hangers-on and get down to the real issue: health.

As we have seen, many of the modern-day diseases can be traced back to what has been called a 'leaky gut'. There are many factors that can erode gut health including chemicals, medicines, diet and stress. Combinations of these are hard to avoid in today's world and if you have any kind of modern-day affliction like obesity, type 2 diabetes or an autoimmune disease then you probably need to repair any damage to your gut before you can see any sign of improvement in your condition.

TOUGH, ROUGH AND SLITHERY: The multifaceted faces of fibre

There is perhaps one magic ingredient that can help heal a damaged gut, increase the production and absorption of vitamins and generally work miracles – soluble fibre. It'll also help you lose weight.

Fibre has various faces. Rough fibres such as wheat bran are way too harsh for the gut. This form of fibre can cause actual harm, just like using coarse sandpaper on a shiny lacquered surface. At the other extreme is the low fibre diet, full of meats and cheeses and eggs with virtually no roughage at all. Such a slithery diet can easily lead to constipation, and if eaten in excessive amounts it can cause kidney disease and weight gain. Such diets are less than ideal. They have a low fibre content and any protein above immediate need is converted to glucose in the liver and stored as fat. We need Goldilocks fibre – something that is just right. This fibre is called soluble fibre and mainly comes from vegetables. If you're a low-GI vegan, this won't be a problem; you'll have adequate vitamins, minerals and a gut microbe fortifying task force of soluble fibre. They love the stuff.

Some scientists think the super abundance of processed foods in the modern diet has reduced the populations of good bacteria in the gut because such foods are deficient in fibre. Study after study has shown that BMI (Body Mass Index) will drop regardless of fat intake if there is sufficient fibre in the diet.

THE SLIPPERY SLOPE TO ILL HEALTH

A low carb diet is often synonymous with low fibre. For instance, many people following the Paleo, ketogenic and Atkins diets think they have *carte blanche* to eat a tonne of meat at each meal. This will of course put their bodies into ketosis and they may well lose weight, but it is probably not the best way forward for optimal health. As the authors of 'The China Study' showed, eating a diet comprised predominantly of vegetables is the most effective way to lose weight, maintain health and prevent chronic disease. It has been shown over and over again that *too much protein in the diet is a good way to ruin your kidneys.* Eating more than 30 per cent protein in your diet makes it too hard for the kidneys to eliminate the ammonia that comes as a by-product of protein consumption. Gout can therefore raise its very painful and ugly head. Later on we will look at Insulin-like Growth Factor 1 (IGF-1) and how too much of it in your body can lead to cancer. High levels are the result of eating too many animal-derived food products. Look into a crystal ball and there's a dialysis machine or cancer in the future of many who habitually over-consume protein, especially animal-sourced protein.

Overconsumption of protein can also result in weight gain. Once the liver converts excess protein into glucose (or lipids), the body has to either use it to power the body or store it as fat. This form of fat is known as visceral fat. It is stored in and around the organs, and because it is metabolically active it is dangerous for our health. Visceral fat acts as if it were another organ by producing hormones like insulin and sex hormones. These extra hormones then interfere with the body's main hormone production areas and result in hormonal imbalances, so you may end up with Polycystic Ovarian Syndrome, Syndrome X, thyroid or gall bladder problems (or, as in my case, all of the above!). It also causes inflammation in the liver and is part of fatty liver syndrome. Where there is inflammation, there is also an immune response involving phagocytes (the immune cells that eat up invading and other unwanted cells). The immune response causes steroid stress hormones such as adrenaline and cortisol to rise. Hormonal chaos ensues.

A rise in stress hormones is often associated with weight gain and fat retention because the body is trying to protect itself against possible negative consequences of the stressor. Stress hormones also have an adverse effect on the thyroid. If the thyroid becomes underactive, the metabolism slows down and the body uses less energy (fewer calories) to carry out the basic processes such as digestion, cell renewal, brain and organ function. Stress hormones also play havoc with the microbiome causing the gut to become leaky and allowing toxins into the bloodstream. This, as we have seen, can cause weight gain and disturbances in mental functioning. All-in-all it's not a pretty picture.

COOKED VERSUS RAW? Who says it has to be one or the other?

Raw food versus cooked food is a bone of contention, but why oh why does it have to be one or the other? There are people out there in blog land who promote diets of raw-food only, but there are very good historical reasons why we cook our food. Over millennia our bodies have actually transformed in response to eating cooked foods: our jaws and teeth are smaller and our guts are quite a lot shorter. It is estimated that our ancestors began cooking food nearly two million years ago. In an interview with Kate Wong for *Scientific American*, anthropologist Richard Wrangham of Harvard University said cooking made food 'softer and easier to digest and thus a richer source of energy. Humans unlike any other animal cannot survive on raw food in the wild. We need to have our food cooked'.

How food is cooked and prepared is also critical to its nutritional value. Some foods actually become more valuable sources of nutrients cooked than when raw. When we cook plant and animal foods we change their chemical structure and by doing so make certain nutrients more easily available. Take the tomato for example, cooking makes the lycopene in tomatoes bio-available and a much more valuable source of nutrition. Asparagus, mushrooms, peppers, spinach, carrots and many other vegetables provide more antioxidants such as carotenoids and ferulic acid when raw. The trick is to not over-cook foods, or cook them at too high a temperature, because doing so can denature the food.

Most plants come with natural defence mechanisms to make them unattractive to various insects or animals. This ensures they are able to reproduce. Some of these chemicals would kill off varieties of gut microbes if eaten raw, but eating them cooked allows us to gain their nutrients without damaging our other gut flora. On the other hand there are plants that put on a pretty negligee of attractive chemicals to ensure they are taken, eaten and spread around by the insects and animals that feed on them.

Once again we find that what was a useful feature in our prehistoric past is now problematic for us. Cooked food provided a more readily digestible form of food and we were able to get a much higher calorie load from it compared to raw foods alone. This was great as it allowed our brains to grow, our intestines to shorten, and it gave us time away from laborious chewing to create the civilised world we now live in. Interestingly however, Rachel Carmody, a former student of Wrangham, showed that mice who ate raw sweet potato actually lost weight compared to those who ate it cooked. Therefore, if you're trying to lose weight, eating a higher proportion of raw food will probably promote weight loss, but including cooked foods in the diet is essential for optimal health.

Having a mixture of raw and cooked foods gives us the best of both worlds.

FASTING: Fasten your seatbelts, you're in for a ride

There are so many different kinds of fasts that it is not possible to cover all of them here. Most people are familiar with the no-food-only-water fast, the juice fast and the intermittent fast. Nowadays the term detox has come to be virtually synonymous with fasting of various kinds, usually with some sort of vitamin and mineral supplementation. No matter what form it takes it is true that fasting has a very long and successful history in every culture and every religion. This fact alone makes fasting worthy of closer attention.

Time and time again studies have shown that fasting makes small animals live longer. Even fasting overnight, or restricting food intake to a window of 8 hours can make all the difference to losing and maintaining weight loss. Intermittent fasting, as it is called, has been shown to have beneficial effects on our microbiome.

The first important effect of fasting we need to look at is its ability to reduce the production of IGF-1, which can lead to cancer if it is too high. According to Dr Michael Mosley, author of The Fast Diet, fasting also switches on some of the genes responsible for repair in the body. He also noted that cancer responds better to prolonged rather than intermittent fasting.

AUTOPHAGY

Autophagy. This odd word appeared one day like a ghost from my days of Latin past. I was watching a TED-X talk on YouTube when it appeared as the title of a suggested video. I read it as auto-phagy and thought, "eat yourself? What the...?"

I soon discovered it was pronounced 'aw-tOff-agy', with the emphasis on the O, but crazily it did actually mean what I thought it meant: eat yourself. It's the body's way of cleaning up metabolic detritus. Cells that are dead, harmful or dysfunctional get eaten by autophagic proteins. The building blocks are then either discarded or reused.

Autophagy is usually set in motion when the body is starved. Most sources I have read recommend a water fast of 4 days or more to set the process in motion. If you have sagging skin or allergies, this could be a solution. I recommend you research the topic and decide whether this is for you. As with any kind of fasting how you break the fast is probably as important as actually doing the fast. Gently ease yourself onto clean, healthy food and keep up the clean, natural fluids while you're at it. And don't have a free-for-all!

Can I recommend an autophagic fast? Not yet. The longest water fast I have ever done was for 3 days, so next time...!

GRAZING ALL DAY? GIVE YOUR GUT A REST

Since the 1980s it has been a popular belief that grazing on food throughout the day activates your metabolism and therefore helps you lose weight. Unfortunately we must buy the burial plot and lay yet another urban myth to rest. Grazing helps you develop high cholesterol, high glucose and liver damage, whereas fasting up to 16 hours a day prevents weight gain, reduces the incidence of liver damage and chronic inflammation along with the diseases that manifest in its presence. This is the case even when the same amount and quality of food is eaten. This means that if you ate the perfect number of calories to help you maintain weight, then eating them as part of an intermittent fast instead of grazing would help you lose weight. Fasting can help combat memory loss as well as diseases like Alzheimer's and dementia.

Basically, you need to give your digestive system a rest so that it can do its job. Part of that job involves moving the food through the body. After two to three hours of being churned in the stomach the food moves into the small intestine where it continues to be pushed through the length of gut by a process called peristalsis. Peristalsis occurs when the muscles of the gut contract in a rhythmic motion, pushing the food (now called chyme – pronounced *kyme*), down the gut toward the anus where it is excreted.

Peristalsis only occurs in tandem with The Migrating Motor Complex, which you will be able to identify as your 'tummy rumbling'. The complex is characterised by waves of electrical activity, and it is these waves that give rise to peristalsis. The Migrating Motor Complex only occurs every 45 to 180 minutes and only when the intestine is given a rest from continual ingestion, that is, between meals when there is a fast of sorts. You will understand from this that grazing all the time isn't such a great idea. If the food doesn't move through your system it stays where it is and that is called constipation. Not fun.

People often wonder why they still need to do bowel movements even if they haven't eaten for a while, or if they've eaten only very little. It may come as a surprise, but up to 40 per cent of your stool is made up of the dead and unwanted microbes from your gut and dead cells from around your body. The average gut microbe lives for about 20 minutes and there are billions of them, so although a single one can't be seen with the naked eye, a huge cache of them doesn't go unnoticed! They have to be moved out of the body to keep us nice and healthy. Rot and decay isn't a good look.

FASTING AND OUR BRAINS

Fasting can also benefit our brains. Fasting mice increased production of a substance called Brain-Derived Neurotropic Factor (BDNF). It stimulates stem cells to become new nerve cells in the part of our brains most related to memory. Rising levels of BDNF also have an anti-depressant effect. For this reason it is believed that fasting could improve mood, too.

Many people believe they can't fast for any length of time because they need to eat at regular intervals. They say that if they don't eat every two hours then they crash and need a pick-me-up. Other people say they start to feel generally unwell. If you eat processed foods, throughout the day, especially those with a high glycaemic index, you set yourself up for the highs and lows related to sugar metabolism. Cravings and sugar crashes will drive you to eat every couple of hours and this is not good for the gut processes that allow you to absorb nutrients and efficiently eliminate waste. As Michael Mosley says, 'The recently propagated idea that we need to graze to avoid a 'blood sugar crash' is a myth.'

If you have already read the chapter on Leaky Gut, you will understand that such crashes are inevitable if you eat a diet high in refined carbohydrates such as biscuits, sandwiches and donuts topped up with a soft drink or other sugared beverages. If you are eating a diet of mostly vegetables with the odd piece of fruit and maybe even a small amount of meat, then you are unlikely to have a problem. Such a regime keeps blood sugar levels steady, the 'good' microbes happy and the mind alert, all of which make it easy to keep even healthier through intermittent fasting. If you avoid carb loading then the crash won't happen. *Lose the highly processed carbs, lose the crash.*

On his fasting days Dr Michael Mosley eats breakfast at 7:30 a.m. and dinner at 7:30 p.m. and nothing in between. This way he gets two fasts into each day and he does this five days a week. In studies that were conducted with mice it was shown that having your first meal at 11 a.m. and your last at 7p.m. is an even better approach. It is always advisable to cease eating at least two hours before going to bed. Personally, because I'm a late night person, I have my first meal at around 1 p.m., my second around 5 p.m. and my last between 8 and 9 p.m. which is a good four hours before I retire for the night. Sometimes I have only two meals instead of three.

Critics of fasting regimes say that it will slow your metabolism, but according to Dr Mosley 'Even extreme fasting – an absolute fast for three consecutive days or on every other day for three weeks – generates no decrease in metabolic rate. Nor does Intermittent Fasting raise levels of the hunger-stimulating hormone ghrelin.'

TO EXERCISE OR NOT TO EXERCISE – that is the question.

Although genetics affects our eating and exercise habits, the environment plays a slightly more important role when it comes to how much energy we expend. We do not lose significant amounts of weight by exercising because our bodies compensate. *The amount of energy we use when we are at rest will stay low or even drop by up to 30 per cent if we exercise too much when trying to lose weight.* So those people out there who think you have to exercise like mad to lose weight, take a word of advice from the professional who has guided many overweight people to a happier, healthier way of living: Dr Sandra Cabot actually advocates against over-exercising during attempts to lose weight. She says that too much exercise can actually stop or slow weight loss. This doesn't mean you shouldn't exercise at all. Far from it. Exercise is important for fitness and general health, so doing about thirty minutes of moderate exercise on a daily basis will keep you in good stead. Once you have reached your goal weight you may want to increase the amount you do to keep you fit and maintain your weight.

Basically, if you try to lose weight mostly by increasing the amount of exercise you do and not by changing sloppy dietary habits, you may find the whole gym shoe experience very demotivating. After putting in all that effort and getting little or no reward you will likely give up on the whole weight-loss gig. Once you realise that what you put in your mouth is the main factor in weight loss, the sooner your motivation to succeed will be rewarded and the smoother your road to weight-loss success will be.

The benefits of exercise are undisputed. What is less clearly understood are the differences between men and women when it comes to exercise. What types of exercise you should do and when you should do it varies depending on your sex. According to studies done by Michael Moseley, 'exercise training in the fasted state is more effective than exercise in the carbohydrate-fed state. This is true for men, but not for women.' A trial on the television documentary series called "Trust Me I'm a Doctor" showed that women lost more weight if they exercised after a meal rather than before. Another interesting fact was that 'fasting women have a better response to endurance training than weight training, while men may fare better with weights.' The concept of sexual equality in nutrition and exercise is a non-starter.

Another major advantage of regular exercise is that it prompts your gut microbes to produce more of a substance called butyrate, which is a short chain fatty acid (SCFA) produced in your gut by the bacteria that live there. SCFAs are essential for healthy gut cells and they play a major role in preventing and repairing a leaky gut and the diseases associated with it such as diabetes and autoimmune disease.

CHEW, BABY, CHEW

We've all been told to chew our food slowly, but in our busy world grabbing a bite to eat often means driving through a fast food outlet and scoffing a burger absent-mindedly while wending our way through traffic or sitting at our work desk. Such unawareness habits are not good for digestion, health or focus either.

When we smell food our bodies prepare for an incoming morsel. We begin to salivate, which is the first step in digestion. Our bodies expect us to take our time with this so it can begin to detect what kind of nutrients are being consumed. This allows the whole digestive system to gear up with the right enzymes and processes to ensure that we get the most from our food. This is also the reason why my preference is to eat calories rather than drink them. I tend to drink water, tea and vegetable broth. A little alcohol occasionally. It is far too easy to over-consume calories when you drink them in the form of juices, smoothies and sodas.

The type of food we eat determines how much we need to chew. The act of chewing seems second nature to us, and most of us speed chew, unaware of how important it is to all the processes that follow. Chewing makes the food softer and mushier so that we can swallow it without choking, but the reason it is so important to chew our food well is to allow the enzymes, (delivered by the saliva) to do their job and partially digest the food before it even reaches our stomachs. It is important to chew carbohydrates well, especially grains, as they take a great deal of effort for the body to digest. If they are not properly pre-digested before reaching the stomach they can create havoc further down the line.

Another problem is that we often choose "no-chew" foods like pasta that deliver their calories straight to the stomach without a backward glance. There is no time for the body to send signals that would see the release of enzymes especially made to digest simple carbohydrates, so when the sugar load hits there is an immediate insulin response and we all know what that means for us: tiredness, a munchies attack in two hours time and a propensity to store those calories as fat.

With repeated hits of chewless food the gut microbes also get out of kilter. They are expecting nutrients from the calories just eaten and when they don't recognise them they force the brain to keep asking for more food. You can see the problem here: the no-chew foods don't keep you satisfied for long and they contribute to overeating. Message: chew your food with awareness. Even if you are on a juice fast, chew your juice!

FRUITS AND FRUCTOSE –
Is fructose really the villain of the piece?

Foods that are too easy to consume and digest contribute to weight gain because their immediate sugar-hit leads to insulin release and subsequent fat storage. Another problematic food that bypasses the normal modes of calorie control is fructose. This comes in some highly delicious, highly nutritious, beautifully packaged combinations such as grapes, pineapples and mangoes! There are several important things to keep in mind when consuming fruit because eating too much or eating it in combination with certain other foods can be problematic.

Firstly, it's important to understand that fructose is a bit of a ghost nutrient. It hides away in the food and doesn't let your body know it's there. Like a 3-D printed weapon it can bypass the normal security mechanisms for detecting calories. The body has ways of knowing how many calories have been consumed and it uses this information to let us know when to stop eating. Unfortunately, this sneaky critter dumps its load on the liver without telling the brain it's doing so. As a result, it's easy to keep on eating. Eating more than the recommended two to three servings of fruit per day can lead to gradual weight gain. You might think you are doing yourself a favour by eating a lot fruit, but too much of a good thing is still too much.

The other problem with fruit is that a lot of people prefer to consume it as a juice. Don't. Well try not to, and not too often. Without all of the fibre that goes into nature's packaging, drinking juice is pretty much the same as drinking a can of soft drink with a few added vitamins plus you've got the added niggle of the fructose doing its magic cloak trick.

The second important thing to keep in mind with fruit is that, if you are eating a diet containing animal protein, it is unwise to eat fruit at the same meal. Many people think they are being virtuous when they have a 'light' fruit salad after a Sunday roast. The trouble is that the fruits will affect the way the meat is broken down and used in the process of digestion. The meat ferments in the intestine causing it to stay there longer and rot. This upsets the microbes and predictably they get a little antsy about this. Upset tummy, anyone?

According to Alanna Collen in her book '10% Human', the fructose in sports drinks encourages growth of the more harmful gut microbes, as it causes fermentation leading to bloating and discomfort. There are better ways to get mental clarity than drinking these industrial chemical concoctions – like having a balanced microbiome and the improved mental health that follows in its wake.

Collen also notes that fructose consumption (in rats) causes toxic changes to the microbiome, leading to fatty liver and the accumulation of visceral fat around the organs. There is a well-documented phenomenon called TOFI – Thin on the Outside, Fat on the Inside. To look at some people you would never guess that they were so metabolically ill and primed for diabetes, heart disease and the like. But there it is, a whole swathe of the population with metabolic disorder who do not have the tell-tale sign of obesity to make them stop in their tracks and take a good look at their diets. Are you one of them?

LET'S GET A TAKE AWAY....

1.
Obesity is not as simple as calories in, calories out. It's your gut microbes that regulate how many calories you absorb from what you eat.

2.
Obesity is not just a personal problem. It is the result of decades of political and commercial misinformation.

3.
Humans are not machines. They are very complicated quantum creatures and every one is different. One thing holds true: the Western diet causes metabolic changes that set us on the road to overweight and ill health. The solution is to reduce processed foods and eat more fresh, whole, plant foods.

4.
Genetic research shows that eating a diet high in processed carbs early in life can switch on the genes for fat storage and lead to obesity in years to come.

5.
Poor gut health prevents the brain from recognising signals from the satiety hormone Leptin.

6.
A diet high in polyunsaturated fats such as margarine and seed oils promotes the growth of bad bacteria in the gut.

7.
Too many of the wrong kind of gut bacteria causes food cravings that are hard to resist. Will power is severely tested when up against biology.

8.

Forget about carb versus protein versus fats. Follow Michael Pollan's mantra: "Eat food. Not too much. Mostly plants." When you do this you can eat to your heart's content and still maintain great health.

9.

Low carb diets are often low in fibre too. The by-products of protein synthesis can lead to kidney damage and painful gout. It can also lead to fatty liver, which is a precursor to metabolic syndrome, type 2 diabetes, pervasive inflammation and the diseases caused by it.

10.

Cooked versus raw is also a non-issue. Do both.

11.

Fasting, especially intermittent fasting is a valuable tool in weight control. It also plays a role in achieving optimal physical and mental health. It does NOT slow your metabolism as claimed.

12.

Exercise while losing weight, but not too much. More than 30 minutes a day of gentle to moderate exercise such as walking can stress the body and prevent weight loss.

13.

Chew your food thoroughly. Don't count it, feel it in your mouth. It is the first step in processing food for optimal benefit.

14.

Fruit is great for you, but be mindful of the amount. Eat it, don't drink it! Fruit is not a guilt-free food. Excess consumption can lead to fatty liver and metabolic disorders including type 2 diabetes.

CHAPTER 4

YOUR FAT PROFILE - NOT ALL FATS ARE CREATED EQUAL

For heaven's sake, get over it! Saturated fat is not a villain. Look at the evidence all around you. All those overweight people (at last count around 60 per cent of the population), well they've probably all been on low fat regimes since the 1970's or 80's, if not longer. And where has it got them? Right where they tried so hard not to be: fat and ill. So just lay off, will you! Let's learn a little about what is really going on in lipid land and get a better perspective.

Saying that saturated fat is not a villain by no means implies that you can go out and eat it to your heart's content. (In fact, your heart would be anything but content!) But what you do need to know is that saturated fats like butter, coconut oil and even lard, are not your enemies unless you eat them by the truckload.

Want a nice case of chronic disease? Try man-made fats like margarines and seed oils (so-called vegetable oils). These are found in products like cheap vegetable oils and margarines. They're a sure fire way to illness.

So let's start at the very beginning: lipids are fats. They come in a fancy-dress ball array of different kinds – all dressed up to impress and in many cases mislead or even outright deceive you, because you don't know who's behind the mask.

Throughout history, eating fat has been part of a diet that helped the human race swing out of the trees, trudge across the savannah and then much more recently climb into motor cars and fly the skies. Without lipids our brain cells and every other cell in our body would cease to exist because the cell membranes that encase our internal engines are made of the stuff – most particularly cholesterol. So you can see that fats are essential to our being.

FATS FATS FATS – so many to choose from

There are saturated, monounsaturated and polyunsaturated fats; long, short and medium chain fatty acids; low, very low and high density cholesterols; omega 3s, 6s and 9s and that's just for the entrée in a world where the sheer mention of fat strikes fear into faint-hearted folk. There's only one piece of advice worth its weight when it comes to fats: if it's natural and made from fruits, nuts or animals, then it probably won't harm you. You'll notice I say "probably" won't harm you. There is a disclaimer: do not overheat your oils. Heating oils above their smoking point transforms even the freshest, healthiest oils into trans fats. Trans fats have a deservedly bad rap sheet. They've been tried, convicted and sent to languish in nutritional purgatory for good reason: they're toxic.

So what kinds of fats are on the healthy menu? How much of them should we eat? What fats in particular should we avoid?

FOR THE LOVE OF LIPIDS

As I mentioned at the start of this book, I used to conscientiously avoid fat – in fact, I was paranoid about consuming fat. It took a lot of reading and research into the latest science to get my head around the fact that I could eat a little fat with a good conscience. When I changed to a low-GI vegan diet I decided I would include "good" fats in my diet and not worry too much about how much I was using. I didn't use massive amounts, but I gave myself a break and let myself enjoy the taste of foods that included fat: avocado, coconut yoghurt and I even cooked with fat! All my blood profiles have improved despite the inclusion of fat in my diet. And I feel great!

SATURATED FATS

The idea of eating animal fats in the form of butter, lard and dripping is pretty much anathema to anyone born after 1950 when we were led to believe that eating saturated fat caused heart disease. This idea now stinks like sheep after a heavy downpour, but it is still pervasive in advertising and the media. Time and again it has been shown that there is no truth to the idea and that the science behind it was more than dodgy, it was wantonly deceptive. In Nina Teicholz' watershed book called "The Big Fat Surprise" she lays bare the anomalous methods used to advance the low fat cause and the lies and deception involved in perpetuating the myth to the advantage of big food companies, lobby groups and the aggrandisement of various scientific egos. A shocking web of lies and deception has caused the nutritional downfall not just of the world's most influential nation but also of all those nations that followed America's lead – basically the whole Western hemisphere and then some.

As a vegan I have not had to contend with this problem on a personal level, but it is troublesome for many people who still believe they have to eat the lean cut of steak rather than the fatty one. Recent studies continually replicate data that show how the lean cut of meat is actually worse for you than other cuts. Firstly, the saturated fat in non-lean meats is not going to harm you unless you eat it by the ton, which is hard because fat is filling. Secondly, the lean cut will not sate you as easily as the fattier one and you may eat more as a result. Thirdly, and most importantly, is the sobering news that the leaner the meat the more L-carnitine it contains.

L-CARNITINE – the good and the bad

So what's this L-carnitine stuff? Well, it is a compound found in animal products – yes, even fish – some energy drinks (where it is added as a supplement), soy and eggs. It helps oxidise fatty acids and is not such a good thing because, in short, it produces free radicals and can contribute to some pretty nasty diseases. L-carnitine is concentrated in muscle tissues, that is, meat. Many readers will recognise the name as a performance-enhancing drug for people keen to build muscle themselves by borrowing it from another animal. But there is a problem with excessive consumption of L-carnitine.

When we eat too much carbohydrate, protein or fat at a meal the body can't use all of the energy right away and so it needs to store it. L-carnitine helps break down the large fat molecules into triglycerides and as we will see elsewhere, this can be severely problematic for our health in many different ways. Basically though, and perhaps a tad too simplistically: too many triglycerides will be stored as visceral fat and can lead to various diseases like diabetes along with all its complications. A high level of triglyceride in your blood test shows that you are probably eating more than you need, especially too much carbohydrate or alcohol.

L-carnitine tends to be a nice guy who is easily led by other troublemakers. When he gets out on the town with certain common gut bacteria like Acinetobacter, he transforms Dr Jekyll into Mr Hyde. You probably wouldn't even recognise him once he turns into TMAO (Triethylamine N-oxide) - a real nasty piece of work. If you have high levels of TMAO in your blood you need to take every measure you can to lower it as there is a very strong, virtually irrefutable link between high levels of TMAO and cardiovascular disease. It's even been implicated in the formation of blood clots, although this is not confirmed, as yet. So keep that meat intake low, preferably zilch.

Clearly the message here is to stay away from meat and animal products as much as possible, and if a wagyu steak comes wagging its tail at you, choose it rather than the pure red, dye-soaked offering of lean meat.

POLYUNSATURATED FATS

These fats were once touted as the saviour of mankind – we were told they didn't clog our arteries like those nasty saturated fats. 'Eat margarine! It will save your life!' Ironically and misleadingly, these are the very fats most likely to get the health authorities' ticks of approval, but as we have already seen, the anti-saturated fat campaign was just so much misguided scumbaggery. We now have convincing evidence that polyunsaturated fats made from grains and seeds like Sunflower seed oil and so-called 'vegetable' oils (usually a blend of any oils that are cheap to produce) are the true villains of the piece.

In the introduction to his book called "Toxic Oils", Australian health crusader David Gillespie notes that cancer, macular degeneration and heart disease can all be laid fairly and squarely at the seed oil door. They may not be the only culprits but with growing certainty they play an insidious role in ill health.

Oxidation is a natural occurrence in the body. Our cells need oxygen, but a vicious circle is continually at play in our bodies. Like a tango partner that repeatedly steps on our toes, the oxygen we would die without also causes damage to the cells it nourishes. This is a natural process and unavoidable, but the consequence is eventual illness and ageing. The body does produce its own antioxidants and we are bombarded with advertising advising us to increase our consumption of pills, potions and palatable foodstuffs to help combat the effects of the oxidative process. However, when we consume polyunsaturated fats in just about every food we buy and eat, they cause an imbalance between the amount of oxidation that takes place and the amount of oxidation the body can handle. This is called oxidative stress.

Polyunsaturated fats readily react with oxygen, more so than other types of fats and they therefore cause more oxidative damage. When the check and balance system is put off kilter by the overconsumption of polyunsaturated fats, things start to go awry and as David Gillespie points out we age faster and we are more likely to succumb to diseases such as cancer, macular degeneration (which is a leading cause of blindness) and cardiovascular disease including heart attacks and aneurysms.

People who follow a paleo diet are doing themselves a huge favour because the diet precludes the consumption of grains. As a result, foods like margarine, which are made from grain seeds, are not part of the food profile. It has been shown that so-called 'healthy whole grains' promote an increase in blood triglycerides, which is dangerous for heart and vascular health and contributes to Syndrome X and type 2 diabetes.

To make matters worse, the way we use polyunsaturated fats make them even more toxic for us. As we saw before, heating oils can very easily turn them into trans fats, which are not found in nature, are totally man-made and do not bond with human cells like natural oils. They don't align with our cells – it's like you've got the right brand of key for a lock but the key won't open it because the profile doesn't match. As a result they cause problems. Even though they are marketed for the purpose of cooking and frying, don't do it. Such pervasive and irresponsible advertising is just more scumbaggery.

OMEGA FATTY ACIDS

Fatty acids come in two types: saturated and unsaturated and they are made up of triglycerides. They are also categorised according to their molecule length. There are long chain, medium chain and short chain fatty acids. They play an important part in gut health. You will have heard of essential fatty acids and you might even recognise some of their names because they are drummed into us by nutritional authorities: omega-3, omega-6 and omega-9, for example. They are called essential fatty acids because our bodies either don't make them or they are not made in sufficient quantities, so we have to include them in our diets.

Omega-3 fatty acids come to us in fatty fish like salmon and mackerel as well as in walnuts, flaxseeds and other plants. Omega-6 crops up in grain and seed products like corn oil, soy, sunflower and other seed oils. It's good to have both omegas 3 and 6 in your diet, but the balance between them is crucial to health.

For most of history the balance between omega-3 and omega-6 fatty acids was about 1:1. Unfortunately we as a society tend to eat way too much omega-6 so the ratio nowadays is more like 6:1. Omega-6 fatty acids are almost unavoidable, especially in the form of wheat, soy and seed products like margarine and oil. They are in just about every processed product you can name; and not just in foods. They are also in personal care products like makeup and toothpaste, skin lotions and shampoos. As a result we are overloaded with omega-6 and this has consequences.

The fine balance between these fatty acids was put out of balance after the industrial revolution when population growth expanded and new technology met the increased demand on food resources by delivering grain-derived products on a grand scale. Mr Kellog in America came up with the cereal flake, which led to the proliferation of breakfast cereals – a true cereal killer! Grain-based vegetable oils replaced animal-based products in the form of oils and margarines and we even started feeding livestock grains instead of grass.

There was a flow-on effect for us - the end consumer. The more omega-6 we ate, the less omega-3 was available to our bodies. Omega-6 is pro-inflammatory and contributes to illnesses such as arthritis, atherosclerosis, allergies and autoimmune diseases, obesity, psychiatric disorders and type 2 diabetes. That's why we're advised to increase our consumption of seafood, especially fatty fish, because it helps counteract the negative effects of too much omega-6. For non-meat eaters there are good sources of omega-3 fatty acids in chia and hemp seeds, linseeds and walnuts. Dr Michael Greger, author of "How Not To Die", says that if you do nothing else to improve your diet, add linseeds, but make sure you grind them first, otherwise the nutrients will pass right through you!

CHOLESTEROL

This old spectre rattles its chains again. As mentioned earlier, cholesterol is the building block for our cells. Only about 20 per cent of what we need comes from our food, the rest is made by our bodies, as is needed. If we eat a lot of cholesterol-containing foods our bodies will tend to make less. There are a few less fortunate souls whose bodies haven't quite got a grip on this and they do have genuine problems with cholesterol consumption, but they are few and far between.

In his book called "Wheat Belly", Dr William Davis states that "cholesterol has little to do with the disease of atherosclerosis". In other words, heart and vascular disease are mostly caused by factors other than a person's cholesterol levels. When discussing cholesterol it is important to understand how the different kinds of cholesterol are synthesised by the body, as what we eat helps determine the proportion of "good" and "bad" types. Scouring food packaging to determine how much cholesterol is in a product is pretty much a waste of time. Your time is much better spent paying attention to total carbohydrate, fat and protein ratios.

My personal view on these things is that if the product you're looking at has to have a label telling you what's in it, then it's probably not actually a real food and is best left on the shelf with the other food-like products. But I do appreciate that occasionally it's nice not to have to make everything you eat from scratch. I do have a way of getting round this difficulty, but you can go to the Eating Upside Down blog for that.

High Density Lipoproteins (HDL) are considered "good". The higher your proportion of HDL to LDL (Low Density Lipoproteins) the less likely you are to have cardiovascular problems. But this is not the whole lipo picture. LDL molecules can be either big and fluffy or small and contained, and it's your diet that determines which kind predominates in your system. All cholesterol starts out as VLDL (Very Low Density Lipoprotein) which then becomes either big or small.

The big molecules are less prone to oxidation, so it is the small ones that tend to cause the problems. Their characteristics enable them to embed themselves in artery walls and cause the build-up of plaque, which, if the diet of highly refined foods continues unabated, can easily lead to blocked arteries. We all know how this scenario pans out: cardiovascular disease including strokes, TIAs and heart attacks. You can usually tell which kind of LDL you have most of by checking out your triglyceride count. The higher it is, the more likely you are to have the smaller LDL that causes traffic jam chaos in your arterial super highways. Reduce the amount of refined, processed foods like bread, pasta, soda, alcohol and biscuits in your diet and not only your lipid profile should improve but your overall health, too.

This factor is particularly important for me because of my family history. Obviously eating habits develop from your family environment and I grew eating way too many high GI carbs like bread, cake and biscuits. As a result I had unhealthy lipid profiles. This led to many of my immediate forebears having aneurysms and vascular disease and they died from strokes, heart attacks and ruptured aortas. When my mother very nearly succumbed to a dissecting aorta I decided it was time to get a grip and take control of what went in my mouth so I could try to avoid a similar demise. I am not fixated on having a long life, but I do want my time on planet Earth to be healthy and full of vitality.

NUT OILS

These oils are best cold-pressed. Once you start eating oils extracted using chemicals and ultra-heat you've lost the battle. For millennia civilizations around the Mediterranean relied on olive oil for many of their daily requirements. It was used in cooking, skin care and cosmetics and lamps to write your parchment by. The olives were simply pressed to extract the oil and then stored in ceramic urns called amphora to protect it from oxidation (that is, to stop it going rancid). Cold-pressed oils are the way to go.

Some nuts are fairly high in omega 6 fats, which can raise inflammation if consumed in excess, so as with many good things in life, choose moderation. Many vegans use nuts to create superb foods that imitate and even surpass the flavour and texture of animal-based products such as cheesecakes and cheeses. A cautionary note here is to keep an eye on the total consumption of nuts. It can be easy to overdo the dose. Remember, foods that are treats are for special occasions, they are not everyday foods, whether they are vegan or not.

If you are eating a vegan diet to reduce your weight try to keep in mind that although sugar and other sweet foods like maple syrup or agave syrup may be a plant products, they really aren't great for weight loss. Low GI is the way to go. Also note that peanuts are not nuts – they are legumes and play a different role in the food landscape from other 'nuts'.

So to answer the questions of which fats are healthy and which to avoid we come back to the sage advice to eat cold-pressed oils made from nuts and fruits. Common oils in this category include, macadamia oil, almond oil, avocado oil, coconut oil, olive oil and hemp oil, butter, lard and other animal fats.

Oils to avoid include any oils made from seeds such as margarines, Canola oil, sunflower oil, cottonseed oil, wheat bran oil, safflower oil, sunflower oil and anything labelled 'vegetable' oil.

You don't need to stress too much about quantity. I didn't and I lost heaps of weight. My lipid profile also improved out of sight. Just use what you need, but don't go overboard. If you eat sufficient fat in your diet you won't crave food as much, which is always a bonus. In addition, every cell in your body will applaud you. So take a bow!

HERE'S OUR TAKE AWAY...

1.
Saturated fats are not bad for you. Oils and fats produced from seeds and those manufactured using heat and chemicals (such as margarine) are extremely unhealthy, even toxic.

2.
If the oil or fat comes from a fruit or nut (or even animals for those non-vegie people amongst us), then it will promote good health.

3.

Excessive consumption of L-carnitine found in animal products, converts to TMAO in the body. High levels of TMAO are strongly linked to heart disease.

4.

Eating too many polyunsaturated fats increases triglyceride levels leading to cancer, macular degeneration and heart disease. These fats are derived from so-called healthy whole grains and seeds and are found in baked goods, margarine and polyunsaturated oils.

5.

Omega fatty acids have to be obtained from the diet. There must be a balance between omega-3 and omega-6. Too much omega-6 is unhealthy. Omega-6 comes predominantly from seeds and seed oils in the diet. Processed foods including bread, margarine and pasta are full of them.

6.

Cholesterol is essential for making each and every cell in the body. Don't be scared of it. Those cholesterol myths are just ghosts of the past.

7.

Eating foods high in cholesterol does not cause high cholesterol in the blood except if eaten in massive amounts. The body produces what it needs. If you eat a lot, then the body produces very little. Only a minute percentage of people have a genetic profile that causes problems with cholesterol.

8.

When cooking with oils, do not overheat them as they will turn into toxic trans fats.

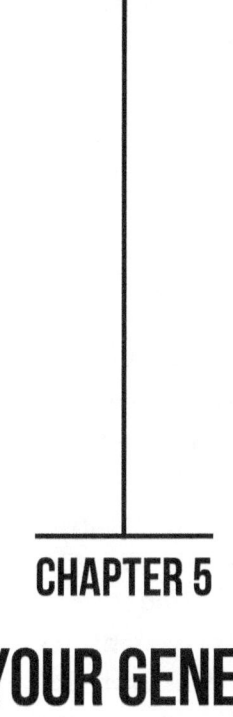

CHAPTER 5

YOUR GENES

The gene genie really is a magical, whimsical entity. So complex, beautiful and radiant that the observer is blinded by his light. He is the shining star in the firmament of medical research. There are so many things we want to know: if only we could pin him down and find the answers to our questions for sure. Why do we get a certain disease and not another? Which diseases is each individual prone to? Can we stave off disease? Is there any way of knowing what we will succumb to, because everyone succumbs to something or other in the end, don't they?

DNA IS A MANY-COMPLICATED THING –
And we thought we'd found the holy grail of health

Just when geneticists think they've got the answer to a question, up pops the genie to confound them again. When scientists discovered that a mutation to the *BRCA1* gene increased the risk of breast cancer, the breakthrough was trumpeted across the world. Finally we had something reliable we could handcuff to a desk and interrogate in depth in the hope of finding a cure. The *BRCA1* gene mutation was determined to be hereditary, which was not good news for all those women out there with mothers, aunts and sisters who had been afflicted by this ugly disease. Interestingly though, research showed that having the mutation did not necessarily mean that you would definitely get breast cancer. There were other factors at play.

As is typical of life on planet Earth, nothing is clear-cut. Everything is connected, whether we are aware of that connection or not. In fact, although we as a species think we know an awful lot, it just ain't true. We actually know very little about life and the universe, and the more we discover, the more we realise that we have only glimpsed the very tip of the scientific iceberg. In the field of genetics we thought that once we had mapped the human genome, and identified all our genes, we would have the answers to all our questions, but in typical gene-genie style our longed-for answers only threw up more and more questions. To our consternation we found that gene X did not necessarily result in disease Y. And why did the rest of the alphabet join in as interlopers to confuse the issue? Did X + A, D and K equal Y? Or did Z hop on board at station P and derail the whole train of events?

EPIGENETICS – The future's in your gut

Some very astute observers sized up the evidence and developed the notion that our environment directly affects whether the genes we inherit are expressed, or not. This idea became an entirely new branch of science called epigenetics. In his seminal work 'The Biology of Belief', cell biologist and epigenetics pioneer Dr Bruce Lipton states that 'environmental influences, including nutrition, stress and emotions, can modify those genes without changing their basic blueprint'. He explains how cell processes at the most microscopic level determine whether our inherited genes are activated or not. Genes are the blueprint, but your life is the construction engineer.

It is crucial to understand that just like an app on your smartphone, a gene has to be turned on for it to have an effect. Some apps run in the background all the time for proper functioning of the phone, others get turned on or off depending on what's happening in the world. Then again, some genes are more like malware that hide away and only come to life in specific circumstances and we usually get a very unpleasant surprise when they do. When it comes down to the line all genes can be affected by our environment.

What do we actually mean by the 'environment'? Well, although we're not necessarily talking weather conditions here, being involved in some meteorological cataclysm could well impact your genes. A farmer trying to survive a prolonged drought in a harsh environment is usually suffering chronic stress, and a business owner whose entire livelihood is left a sodden mess after a flood is likely to suffer acute stress. Traumas that cause stress, from socio-economic deprivation, the unexpected death of a loved one to achieving meteoric success are environmental stressors that can affect the expression of our genes. Exposure to chemicals, medicines, poor nutrition, bullying and burnout all sit at this same banquet table ready to feast on our genome, given half the chance. Stress is such an important guest in this scenario that I am devoting an entire chapter to it later in the book.

WORLD INSIDE A WORLD –
The clandestine existence of alien genes

When it comes to the human organism it might surprise you to learn that how we function genetically isn't just down to the set of genes we inherited from mum and dad (our genome). Like a trillion Trojan horses the microbes we host in every part of our bodies all have their own set of genes that sneakily play out their own scenarios in every facet of our lives.

Our human genes may help determine which microbes our bodies prefer to play host to, but our microbes' genes help define us and our individual characteristics; from our food and exercise preferences, how we digest and absorb our food, what foods we crave or detest, our immune system and what illnesses we fall prey to, our personality and mental health and many other life factors we take for granted.

You can't change your genome, but you can affect how your genes are expressed by paying attention to the foods and medicines you take, your stress levels and your attitude to the world around you. Odd, but true. People debate about whether nature or nurture plays the greatest role in disease, but there is really no contest: it's both. Twin studies have shown again and again that a person can be predisposed to a whole gaggle of genetic mischief makers (nature), but whether or not their dirty tricks develop into a disease comes down to lifestyle and environment (nurture).

In fact, most diseases are not the result of having just one faulty gene that gets activated. This is what makes finding 'a cure' for cancer or 'a cure' for MS so appallingly tricky. There's usually more than one gene at play and for each gene there are probably several factors that cause genetic switches to align thus enabling the disease to take hold. That's a simplistic way of saying that such medical research is fraught with complications. It's not all black and white: there are many shades of grey. No monochrome here.

In her book on "Healing Autoimmune Disease", Dr Sandra Cabot notes that: 'Research shows that 70 to 95 per cent of the risk of developing autoimmune disease comes from your environment, not your genes. By environment we mean your diet, your lifestyle, the chemicals you are exposed to and the emotions you experience......Your genes are not your destiny.' If life were a game of tennis, genes would be the rulebook, but the final outcome of the game would depend on the point-by-point progress of the contestants.

So what turns your genes on or off? Have you really got any control over what happens to you or is life really just a lottery?

QUANTUM EATING – Eating for a whole new world

A landmark longitudinal research project called "The China-Cornell-Oxford Project", better known as "The China Study", was conducted from 1973 to 1975 by a team led by Dr T. Colin Campbell. It surveyed over six thousand people in 65 counties in China. The results gave the authors insight into many facets of nutrition including genetics. It revealed that the foods we eat play a significant role in how our genes are leveraged. A new field of nutrition called nutrigenomics investigates how food and nutrition affect which genes are expressed, how genes influence our food choices, and the way our bodies are able to produce, absorb and use nutrients. The gut and its microbes play an integral role in this.

You know how it is with kids: you want to let them learn how to do something on their own through practical experience, but then, so it's not a demotivating disaster, you really have to help them out, even just a little bit? Well, it's the same with the gut. Even though our gut wants to make vitamins and metabolites and keep us healthy, it really needs our help to get the job done to a degree where it's not a disaster. Everyday modern life is fraught with all manner of lifestyle pitfalls that could easily put us on a path to ill health.

Although our human genes help determine the ability of our guts to function as nature intended, we really need to do three important things to make sure the process doesn't become an unmitigated disaster:

Firstly, we need to be aware of which foods and medicines our good gut microbes like and tolerate so they can thrive and occupy as much gut real estate as possible. If we are not careful in this matter the pathogenic (naughty) bugs will take up residence like loud, dysfunctional neighbours that lob in and spoil the neighbourhood. Eat clean, natural, unprocessed foods as often as possible. Humans have a long, symbiotic relationship with foods from the natural world: that is, ever since time began, we have been able to use plants in our environment to assist the nutritional and medical needs of our bodies. Man-made foods and chemicals, on the other hand, have done nothing but gnaw away at human health and wellbeing for nearly two centuries now.

Secondly, we need to ensure that our hormonal profile is optimal. This can be quite tricky, especially for women, as we tend to be sensitive to foods that mimic natural hormones. The extra load of these wanna-be hormones puts a strain on our already over-taxed systems and cause normal processes to go awry. Dairy, soy and grains are typical culprits. Without overt symptoms like anaphylaxis or rash these substances can wreak metabolic havoc that often goes undetected until we discover PCOS, thyroid, gallbladder or Syndrome X lurking in the vicinity. And yes, I've been there and done all that, but thanks to my low-GI vegan diet I've managed to clear the slate.

The third thing that is absolutely crucial to maintaining optimum genetic expression is stress control. Chronic stress is pervasive in our modern world. Stress hormones negatively impact our microbiome and can cause damage in all parts of the body. They do this by promoting inflammation, which is at the root of most modern diseases. Worst of all, stress contributes to the process that activates the genes we would probably prefer remained dormant: no doubt we'd all prefer to just let them hibernate for good!

Stress can be dramatically reduced by learning to accept yourself, your past and how you are as a person, and by defining and understanding your sphere of influence, so that you don't get overwhelmed by things you have no way of controlling. Practising gratitude, mindfulness, meditation or doing activities that enable you to focus are also helpful in everyday life, whether that's playing an instrument, painting, volunteering or doing yoga, it's all good. Many authorities in nutrition and genetics have edged into swami territory by advocating that people practise mindfulness and focus in their daily lives as way of preventing and healing disease. Have I mastered this? Can I say from personal experience that daily meditation practice will heal? No. For me this area of healing is a work in progress. There are, however, many studies that have shown the unequivocal benefit of such practices.

Ian Gawler is a notable example of how we can use mindfulness and mediative practices to overcome serious disease. Gawler is an Australian who had a malignant cancer that invaded his lymph nodes, pelvis, left lung, mediastinum and which curled his sternum up out of his chest. He cured himself by following an alternative regime that included meditation and positive thinking. The power of mind over matter is a quantum phenomenon that defies everyday logic, but which, with regular and consistent practice, can be harnessed to achieve optimal health. I can highly recommend Ian Gawler's book "Peace of Mind" and Dr Ainslie Meare's book "Relief Without Drugs" for further guidance on this topic. Both are in the Other Resources section of this book.

FACTORY PRESETS AND METHYLATION –
How to go from healthy to sick and back again

Genes are activated through a mechanism called methylation. This is a chemical process and it is greatly influenced by the three factors outlined above. One of the few things you have almost complete control over in your life is what goes into your mouth. Our diet is a primary factor in regulating genes, so it is fortunate we can exert a great deal of control over this area of everyday existence. Public health campaigns have made us aware of the importance of nutrients such as folate, vitamin B12, vitamin D, zinc, methionine and choline, just to name a few. The production and absorption of these metabolites, known as methyl donors, is largely dependent on your diet and, in tandem with that, the health of your microbiome.

As you can imagine, the actual methylation process is immensely complex and, as yet, not completely understood. However, eating your leafy greens and a wide variety of foods, especially plants, will ensure that your body has sufficient supplies of essential nutrients to keep your genes in good repair. The Japanese have a dietary maxim that recommends you eat at least 32 different foods every day. So eating that vegetable curry is a good choice: with about five different vegetables, oil, seven or more spices plus coconut milk, and naan bread with its own cache of ingredients, you're probably consuming about half your daily dose of foods in just one meal alone. Just eating lots of different real foods will cover your needs without you ever having to think about the fine print on the human nutritional charter. It's that simple.

Your average consumer probably tires of being told to eat green, healthy foods. I know many men and women who scoff at a salad because it's 'not proper food'. Well, have Mr Cancer and Mrs Any-Other-Disease-You-Care-To-Mention got news for them! Somehow eating lots of meat is equated with being manly, an important person or being rich, but swamping your daily menu with excessive animal protein is like committing suicide by mouth. Somewhere along the line we have been brainwashed into thinking that eating masses of protein, especially animal protein, is essential to health. It's not.

The one question on everyone's lips when I mention I am vegan is, "Where do you get your protein from?" I can only assume that brainwashing or ignorance is behind this black hole of understanding. Living things are made from protein. Plants are living things, therefore plants contain protein. No great imagination needed here.

Studies show that on a daily basis we really only need about 0.84g (0.3oz) of protein per kilo (2.2lb) weight for men and 0.75g per kilo (0.26oz per 2.2lb) for women. In meat measurements that is about the size of a small rissole per day for women and a medium rissole for men. Most people I know would eat at least two or three times this amount at each meal. More interestingly it has been shown that over-consuming animal protein can be directly linked to the incidence of cancer, but that plant-based proteins do not have the same harmful effects as animal proteins. Increasing your vegetable protein intake and cutting down on animal protein in your diet is one of the best things you can do for your health and the health of the planet.

Protein is only one macronutrient. Fats and carbohydrates make up the balance of our diets. All are essential and all have been considered 'good' or 'bad' at some stage over the past century, depending on the nutritional fashion of the time. From the 1950's until quite recently fat hemlines were way down and carb hemlines were up. Recent research into the effect of these macronutrients on the expression of our genes may change the terrain of the macronutrient landscape yet again.

We have been brainwashed into thinking that low fat diets with their signature overload of processed carbs and polyunsaturated fat products are healthy. Nothing could be further from the truth. Our DNA says so. And it should know – it's been around since humans slithered out of the swamp as aquatic life forms. I am just one of millions of people on the planet whose personal experience of the food pyramid diet has made them sick while trying to get healthy. Dr Sandra Cabot states that a diet higher in fat than what is currently recommended 'increases DNA methylation of the important metabolism regulatory genes resulting in a lower risk of metabolic diseases not just for adults but also for their offspring. The beneficial effects are inherited in subsequent generations.' So eat well now, for the sake of your children and their descendants, too.

The epigenetic notion that acquired traits can be passed on to future generations is especially eye opening. As crazy as it may sound, the children of obese fathers have been shown to have changes in the methylation of their DNA, which in turn leads to them experiencing ill health. Some guys out there might need to look at their diet in this new light before becoming a parent. Just saying.

And this methylation gig is critically important to our health and longevity. Our genes are carefully wrapped in a coat of proteins that coil around the gene providing a shield of protection against chemical attack. In a healthy person, when each cell replicates and splits in two, the DNA is copied exactly in each part. Occasionally there are mistakes in copying the DNA code, but the immune system zooms in on cells that have faulty DNA and disposes of them. If methylation goes wrong, the ends of the genes (telomeres) tend to unravel and expose the DNA to chemical processes that prevent accurate replication of the gene each time it divides. If the immune system is compromised, say by stress, or a poor microbiome, then the faulty cells stay in the body and keep dividing. This is essentially how cancer starts. This, if for no other reason, should be a good reason to check your diet for excess protein, unhealthy fats and processed carbohydrates. While you're at it, check your attitude to all the small things in life that stress you out.

MTHFR Methyltetrahydrofolate-reductase – Yep. It's a real mutant of a thing.

There are some folk out there who have a genetic mutation that negatively impacts methylation. I had never heard of it until I was tested for it. The gene in question controls the production of an enzyme called Methyltetrahydrofolate-reductase. For simplicity's sake let's stick to its more common moniker MTHFR (easy to remember because of what it looks like!!) A person with the MTHFR mutation cannot dispose of some significant toxins and when this happens deficiencies in folate, vitamin B6 and vitamin B12 can develop. As we saw earlier these methyl donors are essential for the proper functioning of the methylation process – switching genes on and off. Consequently, this MTHFR mutation can be the underlying cause of excessive inflammation, heart disease, birth defects and miscarriages.

Dr Ben Lynch, President and CEO of Seeking Health, specialises in MTHFR research. He believes that 'repairing the digestive system and optimizing the flora should be one of the first steps in correcting methylation deficiency'. Again it is shown that taking care of your gut microbes through eating an optimal diet, replete with fresh vegetables that molly coddle the microbiome, can help regulate what we thought was un-regulatable – the expression of our inherited genes. By this stage you won't be surprised to hear me say that a low-GI vegan diet will help take care of this for you, no problems.

Another key player in this genetic chess game is brain-derived neurotrophic factor. Yeah, I know, another mouthful of unpronounceable syllables that get caught in your teeth while chewing them over. Let's christen it BDNF to keep it simple. This little beauty is the building block of cells that make up our brain, skin and retina and it is responsible for regulating the expression of the BDNF gene, so it's kinda important. The gene for producing BDNF has to be turned on through methylation, and as we already know, this is strongly influenced by our dietary habits and exercise. One omega-3 fatty acid that is particularly important here is DHA (Docosahexaenoic acid – thank heavens for abbreviations!). It is found in cold-water foods like fish and algae but the body also produces it from ALA (alpha linoleic acid), which is manufactured by plants, especially flaxseeds, walnuts and pumpkin seeds. If you eat a broad, plant-based diet you won't even have to think about this. All will be right in your BDNF world.

GENES AND THE BATTLE OF THE BULGE – Is your genome a knight in shining armour or is the armour a little tarnished?

Another little bit of info I want to share with you is about starch-processing genes. You will most likely know from the nutritional pariahs of the paleo world that grains and processed carbohydrates weren't always a major part of the human diet. Humans were hunter-gatherers. They ate mainly vegetables gathered from the soils, fields and forests of their immediate environment supplemented by the occasional chunk of meat from a rare successful hunt. About 10,000 years ago people discovered how to maintain a steady food supply by growing grain crops like wheat and rye. The seeds from these crops could be stored for long periods and used to make other long-lasting products like bread (although not the soft fluffy kind we know today). This was a huge bonus to survival. It meant that even if there was a biblical seven-year drought and the obligatory locust plague, the chances of living to see the next sky fall were much higher than in pre-agricultural days.

I love grains. Especially wheat. The texture, the smell, the taste. Heaven. Buns, loaves, biscuits; pretty much anything in that vein were favourites from when I was a baby until quite recently. Even though I always kept to the recommended five servings per day on the food pyramid, it was always that part of the meal I looked forward to the most. It was also the part that left me wanting and craving for more. I have now learned that consuming grains probably played an enormous role in me putting on weight and causing my thyroid to malfunction: two things that go in tandem. When I look back I realise it was probably a factor in my developing the metabolic disorder called Polycystic Ovarian Syndrome (PCOS) as well.

What we didn't know when I was a toddler, but which we do know now, is that certain people really should not eat grains at all. Especially wheat. It was clear from when I was a young child that I didn't tolerate wheat. I grew up on a wheat and sheep farm and every wheat-harvesting season I would come down with one respiratory ailment or another like asthma or bronchitis. In my twenties I underwent a battery of allergy tests and of the thirty-five or so culprits most were grasses: wheat, rye, clover. I was allergic to every grass they tested me for. Because I associated these allergies with asthma, itchy eyes and runny nose I stupidly continued to eat wheat and rye, unaware of the damage I was doing, not just to my gut, but to my whole body, even at a genetic level.

GENES AND STARCHES –
not everyone processes the same foods the same way

I'm going to revisit the chewing versus golloping food debate here, this time in relation to genetics. When we put foods like bread, pasta and potato into our mouths an enzyme in our saliva called amylase begins to break down the starches (carbohydrates) contained in these foods. As you would suspect, there is at least one gene specifically for producing amylase. Depending on which part of the world you live in, you may have plenty of copies of this gene or very few. The more copies of the gene you have, the easier it is for you to digest starches. The easier it is for you to digest the starches, the leaner you will be. The way the carbohydrates are processed has an effect on the composition of the microbiome, and people who aren't well adapted to eating grains tend to gain weight by eating carbohydrate-laden foods. According to Tim Spector in his book "The Diet Myth":

> 'The altered digestion of the starches in maladapted people triggers a change in microbial composition and the production of different fatty acids. This in turn could lead to more rapid increases in insulin on eating starch, which ultimately leads predisposed people to storing more fat. This indicates that some people eating exactly the same bowl of potatoes or pasta will have a greater amount deposited as fat because of the effect of their genes on their microbes. So a potato is not a potato to everyone – to some people that potato, energy-wise, is like a double portion.'

So, if you are one of those people who puts on weight just by looking at a bowl of pasta, either leave the pasta on the shelf or at least make sure you chew it well to get the best effect of the amylase possible. You might also like to make sure that your vitamin D profile is topped up. Studies have shown that people who have trouble digesting gluten-containing foods (grains) are usually low in this vitamin. Vitamin D is also involved in regulating hundreds of our genes, maintaining adequate levels will help keep things chugging along as well as possible. In fact, there are several prominent researchers out there, such as Dr William Davis and Dr David

Perlmutter who maintain that eating grains will negatively impact nutrient levels, which can be problematic right down to gene level.

VITAMIN PEE - and other expensive therapies

Lacking in vitality? Lousy sleep? Skin a bit dull? You think it could be a vitamin deficiency of some kind, so you throw back a few vitamins and minerals and assume all the myth and hype surrounding such products is true and that you'll be back on top in no time. Now and then that's even true. But only now and then. According to many studies (mostly those *not* conducted by the companies associated with selling the product in the first place) all you'll be left with is a dent in your wallet and some pretty pricey pee in the pot!

OMG! How did we ever survive before vitamins were isolated in a laboratory, characterised and then synthetically reproduced so we could buy them dressed up in their swank, come-hither packaging? Well, basically, we ate food; as many different kinds as possible, preferably fresh and in season. Since time immemorial this is how humans survived. Food was our sustenance and our medicine. Our bodies, in fact our genes, adapted to the cycles of life unique to the particular part of the planet we lived on. That's why Japanese are able to obtain high nutrient value from seaweeds whereas Western Europeans, in general, can't; they might consume exotic marine super foods in their breakfast smoothie, but that doesn't mean they are getting nutritional value per gram. How can this be? If we're all human, what's the difference? Interesting you should ask!

You've really got to hand it to those gut microbes; they're a wondrous, versatile bunch of beasties. It's basically because of them that we can process the vitamins, minerals and other nutrients we consume. And they will create the vitamins we don't get from our food, mostly in our own vitamin factory – the gut. There are thousands of different types of microbes living there inside us. Why so many?

Our microbiome plays a significant role in the production, absorption and processing of vitamins, minerals and factors that help regulate gene expression (methylation). Our microbiome and its genes are critical to

85

our nutritional health. What we eat, what we feel and how we experience the world all combine to manipulate the interaction of the microbiome's components. A trauma like the early death of a parent or the unremitting chronic stress of domestic abuse negatively impact our microbiome by flooding our systems with stress hormones. Through a series of processes these life experiences result in genes being expressed or repressed. Either can result in negative health experiences, some of which won't even make themselves noticed until later in life. As Australian genetics professor Dr Craig Hassed noted in his book called "Playing the Genetic Hand Life Dealt You", 'mindfulness – the ability to pay attention, be present and open to moment-by-moment experience – is the most important single life skill we ever develop for these and other reasons.' For an in-depth discussion of how stress and trauma impact our health I thoroughly recommend Gabor Maté's book called, "When the Body Says No".

Some microbes are multi-taskers that take on several duties at once. Then there are others that prefer to focus on one specific task. And don't be fooled into thinking that microbes work in solitary confinement. Many of these guys form a chain gang where they help each other out to get the job done. Indeed, there are some microbes that perform the same function as other microbes, so they can take up the slack or come to the rescue as needed. For instance, if we try out a new food, our microbes might not know exactly what's coming their way, but they will deal with it using their combined skills. If we keep eating that new food, the microbes associated with processing it will become more prevalent in our microbiome. In the future, these foods and others like it will be more easily digested; vitamins and minerals will be more easily extracted and absorbed. If your gut is not in good condition then these fancy processes will come to grief. Any extra vitamins and minerals you consume will just be wasted, because they won't be absorbed. Expensive pee indeed.

WHAT'S FOR TAKE-AWAY?

1.
Your genes are not immutable - they can be turned on and off in a process called methylation. The environment constantly alters the expression of your human genes along with the genes of the microbes living in your

body. What you eat, think and feel, as well as what you are exposed to all play a part in determining which of your genes are expressed.

2.
Your diet, your attitude, your stress levels and your physical environment all contribute to the health of your microbiome. Look after your gut and its microbes. Solution: Keep things simple.

3.
What you eat and what happens to you in your life can change your DNA. These changes can be passed on to future generations via epigenetics.

4.
Minimise what you keep in your surroundings. De-clutter your possessions. Keep only those things you love, use and treasure. Keep them clean and well stored.

5.
Minimise what you worry about. Know your limits. Know your goals. Have routines and stick to them.

6.
Eating mostly whole, fresh, plant foods like low-GI vegans do, can help calm the mind, and re-set the DNA switches that lead to obesity and other illnesses. See Sara Gottfried's books (in the Bibliography) for how to do this.

7.
Avoid processed foods, especially those with grains, added sugars and chemicals. Eating some occasionally won't kill you, but constant consumption can.

8.
You don't need to take lots of supplements if your gut is healthy - just eat a wide variety of plants. Taking supplements when the gut is damaged is a waste of time and money because they won't be absorbed anyway.

CHAPTER 6

YOUR AUTOIMMUNE DISEASE

The Korowai tribe in West Papua still practise cannibalism and are often at war with neighbouring tribes. Barbaric, we think, just as well they're a bit off the beaten tourist track - wouldn't want to come across them on a hungry day in the jungle! Little do most people know that there are millions of people on the planet whose bodies have taken a leaf out of the Korowai handbook - their immune systems are attacking them left, right and centre, ostensibly eating them alive. Worse still, it appears that there is little chance of convincing the troublemakers to dowse the fire and pack away the cauldron.

If you've read this far in the book you will be aware that a growing number of people are struggling with the internal calamity of inflammation, and there appears to be little they can do about it. It seems that someone has thrown petrol on the fire, is fanning the flames and the whole thing is just getting way out of control. Rubbing arthritic joints with anti-inflammatory salves and swallowing pills to stave off the ravages of psoriasis and diabetes seems to be par for the course nowadays. These diseases are the outward signs of civil strife inside the body – the body is at war with itself. When this happens we call it autoimmune disease.

There are scores of autoimmune diseases that we know about: IBS (Irritable Bowel Syndrome), type 1 diabetes, alopecia, multiple sclerosis, celiac disease, Crohn's disease, fibromyalgia, Hashimoto's, lupus: the list goes on. Dr Sandra Cabot says that 'there is not an autoimmune disease that does not have leaky gut as its basis'. Do we see a chink of light at the end of the autoimmune tunnel? Yes, we do!

OPEN SESAME – The proverbial can of worms lifts its lid

If autoimmune diseases have their genesis in a leaky gut, then something can be done about them: heal the leaky gut. We have already looked at how this can be done, and even though it's easy in principle it isn't easy in practice, because most people don't want to change the habits of a lifetime – even if those habits are killing them. We love our vices; they keep us happy and content most of the time, until they get the better of us. No one wants to give up something they see as an enjoyable part of their lifestyle, whether that's having a few beers after work, a bag of crisps in front of the telly or a smoke after sex. It's the little things in life that keep us going, right?

Right at the outset I must tell you that just because you have a leaky gut does not mean that you are bound to get an autoimmune disease. It does however leave you wide open to one, given the right conditions. Similarly, just because you have the gene for a disease doesn't mean you're going to get it. Put the two together, however, and you've got the can opener out and primed to lift the lid on that can of autoimmune worms.

It is curious to note that an autoimmune disease often comes on after a bout of illness; a viral infection like the flu or mononucleosis, or some other stressful situation. Interestingly many autoimmune sufferers have linked the onset of their autoimmune disease to a course of antibiotics. In some way, these are catalysts that pave the way to autoimmune disease. Initially, in a line-up of guilty suspects, it seems fair to point the accusatory finger at the bagman, zonulin, wearing his black hat and guilty face. After all, as we saw in the section on leaky gut, he's the one who causes the tight junctions of the gut lining to ease apart and let the bad guys into the bloodstream, leading to havoc and mayhem. But he's not the only culprit; you are, too.

Yep. Zonulin was nabbed for the crime, but you were the accomplice. As a mitigating factor in your defence we might find that you had a few cronies whispering in your ear at the time of the original offence: suave, sophisticated Mr Anti Biotic and the less salubrious Ms Food Sensitivity, were probably co-conspirators. Together though, you managed to commit a break and enter without alerting the body's defences, and then went on to steal your health in the form of an autoimmune disease.

TAKING CARE OF BUSINESS – the immune system struts its stuff

Immunity cannot be taken for granted. It's not something to be sneezed at. If our immune system is out for the count, so are we.

Together the tissues, cells and organs of the immune system track down and destroy foreign invaders that have no place in the healthy functioning of our bodies. Our sentinels, the white blood cells, patrol throughout the body 24/7. Whether we breathe in a virus or cut ourselves while opening a can, the immune response is to capture and obliterate the intruders. But how does the immune system know which cells to attack and which to leave unmolested?

The body's cunning trick is to employ an array of immune cells like B and T lymphocytes, antibodies and phagocytes that use their combined skills to eliminate invaders. Like a highway patrol car that can detect when an unregistered vehicle drives past, our immune system matches the chemical markers on cells against their checklist of possible invaders. A big job. If an 'unregistered' cell is detected, the system pulls over the offender and deals with him – harshly.

In most people this system works well and we tend get over a cold and heal after surgery. Unfortunately there are several ways things can go wrong, and a leaky gut is one factor that can lead to catastrophic breakdown. Essentially, the software in the immune system's patrol car wrongly identifies passing cells as being foreign, so it ends up tracking down and annihilating not just invaders but the body's own cells as well. This is autoimmune disease, and it can happen to just about any part of the body.

If unwanted substances like endotoxins in the intestine reach the bloodstream via a leaky gut they can cause an immune reaction. The immune system creates an array of agents with fancy names like cytokines, interleukins and interferons. These agents signal to defensive troops who then come storming in to rid the body of intruders. This process results in inflammation, which as we have already seen, is the basis of most modern-day diseases, particularly autoimmune diseases.

To stop this from happening we need to have a gut lining with nice, tight junctions that doesn't let trespassers into the bloodstream. When gut microbes feast on soluble fibre they produce short-chain-fatty-acids (SCFAs) such as butyrate and propionate, which help ensure that the gut lining stays strong. The SCFAs also act in tandem with immune receptors like GPR43 (G-Protein-coupled Receptor 43) to reduce inflammation. Ensuring a good supply of foods high in soluble fibre will promote the production of SCFAs and enhance this anti-inflammatory process. Those clever and ever-so-helpful SCFAs have got a nice little earner happening on the side here too, in that they activate the production of leptin, which reduces appetite and helps you feel full. Keep those vegies on the menu!

THE PATH OF NO RETURN – really?

An immune system in the throes of autoimmune disorder is kind of like Russia under the spell of the mad 'monk' Rasputin, who promised the Tsarina all sorts of miracles, such as healing her haemophiliac son, but who ended up white-anting the Russian monarchy, leading to its eventual collapse. As we have seen, several factors can white ant the gut's integrity and cause the immune system to cave in.

The immune system is there to protect the body and it's pretty miraculous how it goes about its job. But in conditions such as type 1 diabetes, multiple sclerosis and autism, the immune system is out of control. It's got hold of the wrong end of the immunological stick and has taken to beating the proverbial gift horse in the mouth. Destroying components of the body it was sworn to protect is pretty treasonous behaviour and it has dire consequences.

Autoimmune diseases mostly occur when a genetic predisposition is triggered by trauma, heavy metals, a viral illness or a course of antibiotics, such as can happen with type 1 diabetes. Controversially, this same process is thought to lie behind autism spectrum disorders and other psychiatric issues. This will be discussed further in the chapter on mental health. Even severe allergies show that the immune system is out of control. As Tim Spector notes in his book, 'The Diet Myth', children brought up in ultra-hygienic environments, who were not exposed to things like peanut protein while they were in the womb, are more likely to suffer severe allergies. A microbiome that hosts a broad spectrum of microbes is in a better position to support the immune system from the inside out.

There is a significant correlation between various infections and the onset of specific autoimmune diseases. Although Epstein-Barr virus is famous for causing glandular fever (mononucleosis) it has also been implicated in triggering 33 different autoimmune diseases. Another common viral infection, cytomegalovirus has been shown to be a risk factor for multiple sclerosis and Guillain Barré syndrome. Another common virus called norovirus is renowned as a tummy bug that can sink a cruise ship company. Norovirus is linked with Crohn's disease while hepatitis C is associated with Sjögren's syndrome. And they're just the most common examples.

As previously mentioned, if the gut lining is in poor condition, the body will have trouble extracting the vitamins and metabolites needed for optimal functioning, even if supplements are taken. Vitamin D and zinc are especially important in regard to the immune system. If you are low in zinc you may develop small white dots on your fingernails. Taking a supplement can help, but healing the gut will have benefits far beyond improving your zinc profile. Your levels of vitamin D, on the other hand, can be influenced by several factors. Gluten intolerance and a sensitivity to grains in general prevents the body from absorbing vitamin D, zinc and selenium all of which are essential to the proper functioning of the immune system. Getting vitamin D directly from the sun or using a sub-lingual spray is a good step if you have an impaired gut lining.

GLUTEN

In her book called 'Gluten' Dr Sandra Cabot says that 'gluten intolerance reduces the absorption of selenium, as well as zinc absorption, plus gluten intolerant people have higher requirements for selenium. Selenium is needed by your immune system to fight inflammation, infections and cancer, so you do not want to be low in selenium.' She goes on to say that gluten can actually affect which genes are activated and that 'gluten may be the trigger that turns on the wrong genes in your DNA (genome) and this can cause an autoimmune problem to begin or become worse.' Dr Cabot says:

> 'Gluten intolerance can even damage a part of the brain known as the cerebellum and this can cause a gross disturbance of balance and movement (ataxia). This auto-immune ataxia disappears after gluten is removed from the diet.'

If weight gain is a problem for you make sure you are tested for gluten sensitivity, hypothyroidism and Hashimoto's disease. Grains in general, and gluten more specifically, often lie behind an impaired thyroid. If this is the case, the patient may have a slow metabolism, which can lead to weight gain. Dr William Davis in his book 'Wheat Belly' says that leptin, which is an inflammatory cytokine (part of the immune system) controls the thyroid. He states that,

> 'Studies have also shown that elevated triglyceride levels, also a hallmark of too many carbs in the diet, cause leptin resistance. Not a single drug or supplement on the planet can balance leptin levels. But better sleep as well as better dietary choices will do the trick.'

All of the above autoimmune diseases like Sjögren's, Hashimoto's, Guillain Barré and Crohn's are linked to the condition of the immune system, which is in turn linked to the health of the gut. It is imperative to keep your microbiome in good order by eating a diet high in vegetable matter. As shown by The China Study, this is a proven method of creating the best environment for all those unseen microbes that keep you healthy and enjoying life.

TAKE-AWAY

1.

For an autoimmune disease to take hold you need a combination of a leaky gut, a genetic pre-disposition and a catalyst such as a viral infection.

2.

Eating foods that injure the gut such as grains (with their gluten and leptins) provides the right environment for autoimmune diseases to take hold. Avoid foods you are intolerant of, sensitive or allergic to.

3.

Eating lots of different plants, but avoiding grains and dairy, is a sure fire way to heal the gut and feed the "good" microbes in the gut. This will help stave off autoimmune diseases you might be genetically pre-disposed to.

CHAPTER 7

YOUR GUT, YOUR BRAIN AND MENTAL HEALTH

Most of us are under the impression that our brains are in our heads. That's only partly correct. Yeah, we all know the old joke about it being in an entirely different part of the anatomy, but it's not where you'd actually guess. For very good reason, the digestive system has been called 'the second brain'. The enteric nervous system (ENS) is in charge of the gastrointestinal system and oddly enough is loaded with hundreds of millions of neurons, more than your spinal column, and we all know that's a pretty specialised piece of neurological kit. Why would Mother Nature doll up its least pretentious organ with something as highly prized and glamorous as neurons? It's not quite what you would expect for an organ so tainted with the ugliness of the waste process.

GUTS AND OTHER WONDERS

There's a reason we can feel our emotions in our bodies and not just as thoughts in our minds. We are all familiar with goose bumps, butterflies in our stomach, or even gut pain before a major exam or interview. Our head brain and our gut brain are inextricably linked. Some substances used in the head brain, such as the feel-good neurotransmitter serotonin, also have crucial functions in the gut where they control sleep, appetite and sensitivity to pain. In fact, more serotonin is found in the gut than in the brain itself and there are neurons throughout the gastrointestinal tract. Even more astounding is the notion that our gut microbes affect our emotions and therefore also our behaviour. As the aforementioned butterflies will attest, our emotions also affect our guts. They can even change the kinds of metabolites our microbiota produce, which in turn impacts our health. If you're happy, you are more likely to be healthy too. A microbiome in a sad state of health can be reflected in your mood.

Millions of people all over the world are taking SNRIs and SSRIs like Prozac to help with their depression. These potent neurotropic drugs work by altering the way serotonin is processed in the body. I used to take an SNRI but I don't need it any more. My low-GI vegan diet has fixed that up for me. As I said before, being alive is getting cheaper all the time! If you improve the health of your gut, you may be able to eliminate yet another drug from your medicine cabinet. Just make sure you do it under medical supervision, as these drugs are powerful and not to be messed with.

Because the human organism is so complex it's hard to tease apart various parts of the system, label them and say this bit performs this function, while that other bit performs another function. It's just not like that. Everything is connected. For this reason we may not notice that the piece of cake we ate at our niece's birthday party on the weekend is the reason why we felt good then but are feeling low now, a few days later. The time lapse causes a disconnect. But make no mistake, the gut microbes that help produce serotonin have had their birthday cake and are now crying out for more of the same.

YOU ARE WHAT THEY EAT - cravings, addictions and personality

Research has shown that starches and processed carbs are the preferred diet of the gut microbes that produce these feel-good hormones. Mix that with satiating fats and you're onto a winner. That's why we get cravings for hi carb, hi fat foods and reach for the carton of ice cream, the packet of crisps or the toasted cheese sandwich: they all provide our pleasure-seeking microbiota with the foods *they* want. If they don't get it they will make you feel bad until you do what they demand. Once you give in to that Tim-Tam or burger, you just magically start to feel better again – and so the vicious circle goes round on its merry way. Giving into your desire is not a sign that you are a repugnant, weak-willed person who is slovenly and worthless. Food cravings are a sign that your gut and your brain are having a good old chinwag about what should be on the menu – for them.

Many people who crave processed carbohydrates and starches tend to have major fluctuations in their mood, and it is seen time and again, that people with mood disorders like schizophrenia and bipolar or even a diagnosis on the autism spectrum, often have a major predilection for these same foods. This is no coincidence. The gut microbes that want hot chips for breakfast, lunch and dinner usually get their way because they have taken over large chunks of gastrointestinal real estate and there is no one to oppose them or even ask them nicely if they could try something else for a change. Like peasants after the Black Death who took over farms left vacant by the rapid and unexpected demise of their lordships, these microbes start pushing their weight around. They don't want to be told what to do any more; they're no longer serfs beholden to the masters of the land. They'll have what they want, thank you very much. For this reason changing what you eat to mainly plant-based, low-GI foods may be hard in the initial stages, because by day 3, 4 or 5 the microbes are getting pretty upset – they may even throw a tantrum demanding you feed them what they want. But like a parent that doesn't give in to a child slamming its fists on the supermarket floor, the microbes will come to understand that you are not giving in and will eventually calm down.

CRAVINGS AND ADDICTIONS

Sometimes it's really hard to resist certain cravings. There is even a name for the behaviour of acting like a target-seeking missile headed for the fridge: hedonic eating. This behaviour is intricately bound to the reward system – you know the one where athletes will run through pain just to get their dopamine hit, while others will sell everything they own for the high of ice or cocaine. Oddly enough, people who are addicted to food will gain control over their eating behaviour when given the drug used by alcoholics to stop their addiction to alcohol. This underscores the idea that food addiction and any other kind of addiction are tied to the dopamine reward system. Gut bacteria that cause damage to the gut wall are usually of the Firmicute variety. They make the gut wall permeable and in doing so let through the metabolites that hijack the reward system and cause cravings, binges and hedonic eating behaviour.

Although my cravings for certain foods have not entirely disappeared I can honestly say that my ability to withstand the cravings is very strong. Hedonic eating is a thing of the past. I also have improved mental clarity – the brain fog brought on by a dysfunctional gut and eating foods containing processed grains has lifted. To paraphrase an old song, "I can see clearly now the grain has gone!" If you had told me years ago that all this agonising behaviour was caused by the microbes in my gut I probably wouldn't have believed you. Only recently have scientists been able to use state-of-the-art research methods to show this really is the case.

Dr Emeran Mayer, a forty-year veteran of brain-body interaction research at the Digestive Diseases Research Center at the University of California at Los Angeles has shone a light on the intricate connections and communication between the brain, the gut and the microbiome. As he says in his book "The Mind-Gut Connection",

> 'In a recent study of individuals suffering from alcohol dependence, it was shown that cravings for alcohol during periods of abstinence were positively correlated with the individual's intestinal permeability (how leaky their guts were) and with changes in the gut microbiota.... Given the strong engagement of the brain's stress response during craving and the well-known effects of stress on gut permeability, it's conceivable that the permeability effects in this study were related to a craving-related (and stress-related) increase in the gut's leakiness and the observed

changes in gut microbial composition and metabolic function.'

In more everyday speak this means that the intricate connection between the mind and the gut may be responsible for more than just moods and craving. When combined with a genetic predisposition it may actually lie at the heart of addiction. Studies have shown that the short-chain-fatty-acid called butyrate is a key player in the communication system between the head brain and the gut brain. Butyrate is created by microbes that thrive on soluble fibre so once again the best thing you can do about this is to sway the balance of the microbiome from a predominantly Firmicute environment to a predominantly Bacteroidetes environment. How? Eat mainly unprocessed, plant-based foods.

TREATING THE UNTREATABLE – autism, bi-polar, schizophrenia, MS and Parkinson's – a suite of not-so-sweets

Those not so cute Firmicute bacteria, such as Clostridium (the family that tetanus and botulism belong to) like refined carbs and tend to predominate in the guts of people with mental health problems and neurological conditions. In fact, Alanna Collen's research has revealed that 'compared with [the] healthy children, [the] autistic children had, on average, ten times the numbers of clostridia in their guts.' These bacteria don't like oxygen, so they can thrive in conditions many other bacteria would perish in. That also makes them dangerous, as they are pretty hard to keep under control or get rid of.

Clostridium infections can be treated with antibiotics, but this solution is also fraught with problems, because antibiotics generally annihilate the friendly bacteria too and leave even more room for the bad, pathogenic bacteria to multiply in the gut. That's why, during and after taking a course of antibiotics, it is wise to consume predominantly prebiotic foods (vegetables high in soluble fibre) to encourage the proliferation of 'good' bacteria, and probiotics to re-establish colonies of 'good' bacteria that many have been decimated by the antibiotics.

It's crazy to expect your health to improve if you haven't changed the habits that caused the problem in the first place. How much longer will we continue to follow dietary guidelines that just don't work and which are actually harmful for many people? If we keep bowing to the will of gut microbes that thrive on the modern Western diet of highly refined carbs and seed oils, we will continue to succumb to modern-day diseases. Inflammation-causing cytokines produced by the immune system can cross over into the bloodstream and affect the brain, our mental well-being and our overall health. One thing that can definitely help in the fight against such bacteria, and their desire for the processed starches and carbohydrate-rich foods that pilot the microbiome into never-never land, is a plant-based diet and a low-GI one at that. Taking steps to control the release of stress hormones that also favour the proliferation of these microbes is also a good idea.

As has been previously noted, antibiotics are an essential weapon in the arsenal against diseases that have blighted mankind since time immemorial. Even just 100 years ago a scratch from a rose bush while pruning could easily have killed you. Nowadays it's not so much infections that will get you, but chronic modern-day ailments like diabetes and autoimmune diseases. Antibiotics have been miraculous, but they also have their dark side. In her book '10% Human', Alanna Collen remarks that,

> 'The link between more ear infections and more antibiotics bears up. An epidemiological study showed kids with autism tend to have been given three times more antibiotics than those without it. Those getting antibiotics under the age of eighteen months appear to be at greatest risk… It turns out that 93 per cent of children with autism had ear infections before they turned two, compared with 57 per cent of children without the condition.'

Although this evidence is not conclusive, it certainly seems to be pointing to a likely culprit. The message is, of course, to be discerning when it comes to the use of antibiotics as they can set in motion the conditions that lead to a leaky gut and its consequences, including mental illness.

GAPS AND PSYCHOLOGY SYNDROME

If someone told you that a severe affliction such as schizophrenia were caused by what many medicos see as a phantom condition – a leaky gut – then you too would probably laugh them out of court. But respected clinician Dr Natasha Campbell-McBride and her colleagues at The Cambridge Nutrition Clinic have developed what is called the GAPS (Gut and Psychology Syndrome) protocol. The science behind this dietary regime reveals that disorders such as bipolar, autism and schizophrenia can be alleviated, not with medicines, but by healing a leaky gut.

Dr Dohan from Community Hospital South and Johnson Memorial Hospital in Indiana points out that schizophrenics tend to have gut problems, whether that is simple bloating or painful Irritable Bowel Syndrome (IBS). His research has shown that the symptoms could be relieved by eliminating grains from the diet. This is quite a big ask for schizophrenics and patients on the autism spectrum as they tend to have a predominance of Firmicute bacteria in their guts that drive them to eat carb-laden, grain-based processed foods. This exacerbates the problems and perpetuates the affliction.

Dr Campbell-McBride quotes Dr J Robert Cade from the University of Florida as saying, "We think that with autism and schizophrenia the basic disorder is in the intestine and these individuals are absorbing beta-casomorphon-7 that they normally should break down in the body as amino acids'. In other words, the microbiome of these patients is impaired and their gut is allowing large, inflammation-causing molecules (in this case from dairy) through the gut barrier into the bloodstream giving it direct access to the brain. The inordinate number of immune cells in the lymph nodes of autistic children substantiates this claim. It shows that they are fighting chronic inflammation.

As we have already seen, such chronic inflammation has an impaired gut lining as its root cause. Throughout this book we have seen that an impaired gut can lead to chronic inflammation. The GAPS dietary protocol used at the Cambridge clinic has had astounding results in treating an array of psychological disorders that mainstream medicine believed were only treatable with potent psychotropic medicines – recovery was never on the radar – it was more a matter of treat the symptoms, not the cause, even though some of the cures made the symptoms worse, not better!

TRANSPOO-WHAT THE?

Apart from following a diet to repair the gut lining there is another new treatment for leaky gut that will have you either laughing, spewing or jumping with excitement. It has been given various names, but my favourite is 'transpoosition'. What is it, and why would anyone really go through with it?

Well, it is technically referred to as a faecal transplant which means taking the poo from a lean, healthy individual and transferring it into the gut of someone who, for whatever reason, needs a repaired microbiome. Doctors in the US, Israel, Australia and elsewhere have had amazing success with this highly unusual and somewhat off-putting procedure. But if you had a bad case of the potentially lethal *Clostridium difficle (C. diff.)*that didn't respond to antibiotics, you would probably choose a transpoosition without hesitation.

At the Centre for Digestive Diseases in Sydney, Australia, a full 80 per cent of patients presenting with IBS due to *Clostridium difficile* infections have been cured using transpoositions. Professor Tom Borody has also had patients make remarkable recoveries from diseases thought to be untreatable, such as MS, Parkinson's and a more obscure ailment called 'ideopathic thrombocytopenia purpura'. Like his colleagues at the clinic in Cambridge, Dr Borody has also had success improving symptoms in autistic children by healing the gut, albeit with faecal transplants rather than dietary intervention.

Australian geneticist, Dr Craig Hassed of Monash University in Melbourne, tells us that nutrition-induced epigenetic changes can alter the risk for schizophrenia and can also lead to disorders like Parkinson's, MS, mood disorders and addictions. The link between what we eat, our microbiome and our mental health has been firmly established. All these afflictions seem to have been tossed into one giant cauldron of roiling intestinal malcontent. When it comes down to it, if we want to avoid the ravages of these common mental and physical diseases we really need to take our diet and our susceptibility to stress in hand, and not let ourselves be lured into thinking that we can eat the standard Western diet, and live the standard Western lifestyle like most regular Western people and not succumb to some sort of Western disease. Keith Richards might have managed it, but who knows what planet he's really from!

HERE'S OUR TAKE AWAY ....

1.

The gut has a direct link to the brain via the vagus nerve, which is part of the Enteric Nervous System. Because of this, our physical and mental health are also directly linked.

2.

The gut produces more neurotransmitters than the brain. These neurotransmitters are crucial to our mental health, so it is important to keep the gut super healthy. Eating plenty of plants and avoiding grains and dairy promotes gut health.

3.

You are what your microbes eat. Microbes that come to dominate in the gut as a result of a diet full of processed foods demand more of the same. You can become hooked on foods that aren't good for you because of this. They will cause you to have cravings. They even cause addictions.

4.

Illnesses such as autism, bi-polar, schizophrenia, MS and Parkinson's, have all been successfully treated by healing the gut. Once again, eating lots of different plant foods and avoiding dairy and grains in the diet will heal the gut and lead to better mental health.

5.

Recent advances in treating gut problems include introducing the gut microbes from healthy individuals into ill people. These faecal transplants (transpoositions) have also helped reverse autism and successfully treat diseases once thought untreatable.

CHAPTER 8

YOUR STRESS LEVELS

Stress is a word that gets bandied about a lot. It's used as an excuse, a blow-softener and a diagnosis. Most importantly, it's real. A long time ago the word stress meant hardship and adversity but a couple of centuries ago engineers used it to describe adverse conditions that led to metal becoming brittle and fracturing under strain. Not long after that, psychologists kidnapped the word and used it to describe a psychological version of the same phenomenon.

In the nineteenth century steel barons were trying to create ever-harder types of steel for their expanding markets. For good business their steel had to be a reliable product. Unfortunately there were mishaps. What made something as strong as steel fracture and cause buildings to collapse and ships to sink? The usual culprit was extreme pressure centred on a localised point causing small imperfections in the steel to give way. It's not much of a stretch to see how this could easily be applied to the human condition. Everyone has a weak spot. Apply excess pressure to the weak spot and the person will give way. What processes actually cause that to happen?

CYCLONE PROOF VERSUS THE HOUSE OF CARDS -
It's all in the manufacture

No two people will react to the same situation in the same way. For some people a harsh comment will be like water off a duck's back while others will take it to heart. How we respond to events in our lives depends on our physical and psychological resilience, and how we perceive our own peculiar set of life circumstances at the time of the event. Trying to understand how and why we react the way we do has filled thousands of volumes over the years, but it comes down to our two favourite old chestnuts: nature and nurture.

Stress has always been a part of the human condition and consequently our predisposition to stress and how we deal with it begins in the womb. Genes are certain to play a role. What our mothers ate and felt while they were pregnant plays a role. What happens to us and how we are treated, especially in our early years, also moulds our ability to withstand stress and trauma.

Stress is another of our ancient body programs that causes us grief in the modern age – it's a weapon that used to enable our physical survival in a perilous and unpredictable world, but which has now been turned against us. Times change quickly, but our genome doesn't. It wasn't that long ago in the evolutionary scheme of things that humans regularly appeared on the menu of some carnivore or other. Nowadays the predators are more likely to be from a corporate jungle rather than one with a treescape, but the effect on us is the same.

NIGGLES AND SLEDGEHAMMERS

Not having a roof over your head, relying on a cache of part-time jobs for income, or not knowing where your next meal will come from are all extreme stressors, but there are other things about modern life that can do us over. Relationships usually top the list along with work pressures and time constraints. Trying to lead the perfect, well-balanced life remains elusive for most mere mortals. It doesn't stop us from trying though! Our capitalist, consumer society is greatly to blame for producing unreal expectations – goading us on and making us believe that we need to buy this or do that to be a worthy human being.

As recently as 50 or 60 years ago, we made do with a lot less; gender roles were rarely questioned and people knew pretty much what life held in store for them: the man provided and the woman looked after the family. Society was designed so that families could live off one wage. Try getting a family of four with a mortgage to live off one average wage now! I'm in no way lamenting the past because it was certainly less than ideal, but the wide landscape of our possible futures is a lot less certain than that of our immediate forebears, and some pretty steep and bumpy terrain lies ahead. Thanks to technology our lives move at an ever-increasing pace. Put all these things together and life has become a bit of a blur. Stressors of all kinds from a multitude of little niggles to proverbial sledgehammers surround us at every turn and make dealing with stress anything but easy.

STRESS SOUP –
A recipe for disaster brought to you by modern life

When we are stressed our bodies release a number of chemicals, some of which are steroid hormones. For thousands of years they were absolutely essential to our survival. Back then, stress usually arose and we dealt with it or got eaten. But nowadays, stress is like Mohammed Ali in a world title fight, it just won't back off.

Modern man is plagued by disorders brought on by the constant release of stress hormones; we suffer anxiety, depression, metabolic syndrome and diabetes, just to name a few. Repeated doses of steroids are extremely detrimental to our health; they destroy the balance of the microbiome and contribute to a leaky gut - and we know the kinds of ailments that arise from an impaired gut microbiome. Gotta hand it to those steroids, they sure know how to party – at our expense!

Our stress hormones might be having a good time feasting away on our microbiome, but how are we doing? We can measure how well we are coping with stress by measuring cortisol and adrenaline levels in our blood. The overall result is known as the 'allostatic load'. We may not realise it, but even things like infections, surgery, accidents and going on a diet are perceived as stress by our bodies and they elicit a stress response. These are the sorts of things that occur in our lives on a regular basis, but if our bodies are producing excess cortisol on such a regular basis we are in for a rough ride. All sorts of things can go wrong from vision loss, to having a compromised immune system, metabolic disorders and memory loss. Stress hormones can interfere with sex hormones and have a negative impact on the reproductive system, too. Adrenal fatigue is becoming more and more common. And these are just the players that have been short-listed for the 'Worst Possible Outcome' award.

Stress hormones have played hardball with my sight and that is why I really have to get my stress levels under control. You could have knocked me over with a feather when the ophthalmologist explained to me that the Central Serous Retinopathy compromising my eye health was brought on by extreme stress. There was only one thing for it – get it under control using meditation and mindfulness techniques. As I write, this is proving harder to work into my lifestyle than any other thing I have ever tried. If you suffer from stress, be aware that it may be causing you more trouble than a missed night's sleep or a few grey hairs. For ideas on what stress can do to you and how to deal with it, go to my blog at eating.upside.down. com and check the section on stress.

MOTHER NATURE CAN BE A RIGHT ROYAL PAIN IN THE GUT

Even before we are born our genes can propel us into a realm of sensitivity others cannot begin to imagine. Just look at a group of toddlers and even at that age you will immediately be aware that there are leaders, carers, bullies and the bullied. How do these traits become noticeable so early on in life? If our parents or grandparents were traumatised through war, famine or family dysfunction, then epigenetic changes in their bodies may well have been passed on to us leaving us vulnerable to stress. Even if none of these terrible life events happens to us personally, our bodies will have the protective machinery in place in case it does – a kind of pre-emptive strike force of genetic soldiers, that plays out as personality traits right from the get-go.

If we have inherited genes that predispose us to sensitivity, nervousness, anxiety and introversion, then poor parenting, bullying and even parents favouring other siblings can cause these genes to be expressed. As a result, we can react to events that would leave other people emotionally untouched. Others may even call us 'oversensitive' and be derogatory about how we deal with things, just because we aren't as gung-ho or confident as they are. Of course, this only makes the situation worse.

I had an acquaintance whose husband, a war veteran, suffered badly from nerves and who was quite ineffectual in the presence of his overwhelming wife, who bullied him mercilessly for any perceived shortcomings. (And continues to do so even though he has been dead for 2 years!) One day the acquaintance was belittling her husband saying he was weak and useless when another friend pointed out to her that he may suffer anxiety to which she replied, 'What's he got to be nervous about?!!!!' Not for one moment did she contemplate that it was her behaviour that exacerbated what was already a character trait inherited and compounded by his time as a soldier who saw active service overseas. Behaviour, such as relentless harassment, turns on the cortisol taps and leaves them to run day in, day out.

DAILY LIFE HAS A LOT TO ANSWER FOR

Ever felt like your brain takes a holiday when a cascade of uninvited guests turn up: the car breaks down, little Johnny catches a cold, the sink gets blocked and the ATM swallows your card? At times like these a hormone in the body called CRF (corticotropin-releasing factor) is secreted in the hypothalamus (the part of the brain responsible for memory) and in the T-lymphocytes (which are part of the immune system) in response to stress. It's part of the reason why we become forgetful when under duress: CRF is blocking the stairs so our memories can't descend! Excessive levels of CRF are just not good for us. If you ever needed a reason to overhaul the hectic lifestyle schedule that stops you from eating, exercising and relating properly then this is it: excess CRF is clearly associated with Alzheimer's and major depression. So grab the big, black texta and slash a few things off that to-do list or schedule!

You have to actually prioritise activities in your life. (You've probably already glimpsed an armour-clad mini-lecture coming round the corner on a high horse here!) There are basically three kinds of people: those who are *pro-active* in their lives, who regularly evaluate their progress, pre-empt trouble and take control to keep on top of things. Then there are the ones who delude themselves into thinking they're in control by being constantly active; they believe rushing around and fitting loads of activities into their day is actually being on top of things. Then there are the *reactive* folks who let life dictate what they do and they feel trampled at every turn. Everyone's a bit of a mix, but you will probably identify with one style more than another. Take a step back. If life is dictating to you and you feel that you are being propelled by some invisible force, then you really need to stop and take stock. Talk to people about problems and find solutions, write it down and review it, keep a diary or calendar and actually use it.

What do you really want from life? No doubt you want health, happiness and prosperity for you and your family. So how does being sick, tired and angry from the relentless chain of stressful chores and misadventures really help you achieve that? The more you stress, the less likely it is that your life will ever be the way you want it to be. Your life and your health are dictated by what you do *most* of the time, so *most* of the time you need to prioritise the food and meals you and your family eat because that is the most important thing you can do for your health and the health of your loved ones. Wherever you can, **simplify.**

If you do nothing else, taking the time to eat well is the one thing that will change your life for the better.

Yes, it takes some planning and preparation and there are suggestions for how to do this on the 'Eating Upside Down' blog, but some things will just have to move down or shuffle off your list of priorities. Preparing a healthy meal is more work than driving through a take-away joint, but if that style of living isn't helping you meet your life goals then you need to change it before you have no choice. What good are all those extracurricular activities doing if you're setting your kids up for the negative consequences of the quick, on-the-run Western diet that so many families give in to? If you and your family are healthy, then those other things will find their place on the planner in good time, and your mind and body will be in good shape to support you in making decisions about your life. Here endeth the mini-lecture.

PAC-MAN INCARNATE – chomping away at your health

When stress hormones flood your body unabated they can cause permanent damage. If you're not careful, all those unprioritised daily lifestyle choices will band together and gang up on you in the alleyway. Together they form what is called the allostatic load and if you're loaded to the brim with stress then health problems will arise sooner or later. Like a jack-in-the-box, once they have made their appearance they are mighty hard to repress and close the lid on – they'll keep rearing their heads again, time after time. The higher the allostatic load the shorter the ends of our DNA - our telomeres. Amongst other things, shortened telomeres can cause depression, ageing and a shortened life span. Interestingly, the more stress a woman is under while pregnant, the shorter the telomere length in her child. The baby can then be predisposed to all the things that shortened telomeres invite, such as introversion (not necessarily a bad thing), depression and general failure to thrive. Even cancer. Stress is one of the main things that will cause telomeres to shorten.

Chronic stress is like a trick-or-treater dressed up as the devil for Halloween. It will roam far and wide collecting sugar treats and creating metabolic havoc. In women it can lead to a deficiency in the sex hormone progesterone that can then cause menstrual problems like PMT and increase the chances of developing endometriosis and uterine fibroids. As if that weren't critical enough, it can also help raise the blood sugar profile and exacerbate the symptoms of PCOS, Syndrome X and type 2 diabetes.

Our modern lifestyles are leaving us open to the negative consequences of stress hormones. An astounding number of people seem to run on caffeine, hi-carb shots and the stress hormone adrenaline. Unrelenting stress can permanently damage the microbiome leading to leaky gut and all of the problems related to it: weight gain, mood disorders, autoimmune and heart disease, to name a few.

Recent research by Professor Herbert Herzog and his team at the Garvan Institute of Medical Research in Melbourne, Australia, has identified a neuropeptide called NPY, which is produced when the body is stressed for long periods. It's been shown in animal studies that NPY is directly linked to weight gain, so that's another reason why it's massively important to keep your stress under control.

SLEEPING IN A GALE – the adverse winds of stress hormones

Stress is also one of the leading causes of poor sleep. Not being able to shut off thoughts about work, deadlines, relationships, family and financial problems brews up a storm that blows through our minds even into the wee hours, making it difficult to get to sleep and stay asleep. Sleep studies have conclusively shown that sleep deprivation causes weight gain. The body sees lack of sleep as stress and, you guessed it, the body responds by releasing stress hormones that cause weight gain and impair the gut and microbiome.

Meditation, mindfulness and other practices that strengthen the mind-body connection have been shown to soften the blow of stress steroids by reducing inflammation. Crucially though, you will need to practise on a daily basis for at least 6 months before change can be measurably noticed. If you're a couch potato and decide you want to run a marathon to improve your fitness, just buying the shoes and heading out on the street won't help you get across a finish line any time soon: you have to train and build up to it – maybe enter a few fun runs and half-marathons first. Likewise, doing the odd bit of yoga or meditation here or there won't make much difference to your overall stress levels or the problems that arise from them. Consistent practise, even for 15 to 30 minutes a day will however make a difference. A big one. It'll give you a podium finish in a matter of months and when you look back you'll think the time it took was nothing in the long run.

The microbes in your gut are working on you around the clock. They produce a neurotransmitter called GABA (gamma-Aminobutyric acid) which helps keep you calm and contributes to a good night's sleep. In addition to this, serotonin is produced in the intestine and gut microbes contribute to the production of the sleep-regulating hormone melatonin. Tryptophan, the crucial precursor to melatonin, is a by-product of microbial action in the gut. So, as you can deduce, a dysfunctional gut can easily play hardball with your stress hormones and hit a home run against you even while you sleep. The bad news on top of the bad news is that poor quality sleep and shorter telomere length go hand in hand which means that you age faster. The meat eaters out there in ignore-it-and-it-will-go-away land may not want to hear this, but a diet high in meat (red more so than white) is associated with shorter telomeres. It's kind of like karmic revenge for the eaten animal.

THE FEEDING CENTRE – How many cells does it take to keep you trim? Fewer than you might think.

In 1998 brain scientists identified a part of the brain they called the "feeding centre". It's a very small part of the hypothalamus and is made up of just a few cells, but do those cells pack a punch! It is responsible not only for appetite but also for sleep. Researchers observed that narcoleptics (people who are unable to control their sleep) were more likely to be obese even though they ate much less than the average person.

It turns out that the feeding centre is actually the master switch for determining our metabolic rate. How well we sleep directly affects how well our metabolism functions and how we use and store calories. If you are sleep-deprived you use 10 per cent fewer calories just to stay alive. If your average daily need is 2000 calories then that's 200 less that you need. Makes a difference!

So ask yourself, do you really want to play with your shiny electronic gadgetry into the wee hours at the expense of your waistline and health? Your choice. If it's an addiction, take it in hand. Make sure you get sufficient sleep. Prioritise!

LIFT YOUR GAME –
but don't strain yourself while you're doing it

Media, and particularly television reality shows, that portray contestants doing mammoth amounts of exercise, hauling trucks and traversing army training courses, have led the general public to believe that in order to shift large amounts of weight you have to do large amounts of exercise. This is wrong. Dr Michael Mosley, Dr Sandra Cabot and many other leading experts tell us again and again that *too much exercise will actually prevent you from losing weight*. Don't get me wrong, exercise is an essential part of a healthy lifestyle, but too much of it is not a good thing, especially in the weight loss phase. As Dr Sandra Cabot states in her book 'Healing Autoimmune Disease',

> 'Exercise that is too intense or of too long duration can also act like a stress to your body by promoting high cortisol secretion. ... It is also best to not exercise for longer than 30 minutes at a time, as this will also help to prevent the exercise from being overly stressful to your body.'

That's it in a nutshell. Couldn't have said it better myself.

TAKE-AWAY TIME

1.
Stress can be brought on by modern life. Not having a steady job, living in crowded, noisy cities, eating processed foods, over exercising, relationship problems, too much to do in too little time.... the list goes on.

2.
Getting your stress under control is essential for good health. Your level of stress and your stress coping mechanisms dramatically impact your health for good or bad. Meditation and any other mindfulness practices are essential. You'll be healthier, make calmer, more focussed decisions, and you'll be easier to live with!

3.

Our bodies release stress hormones when stressed. These are perfect for the occasional one-off situation, but chronic, on-going stress is damaging. Stress maims your gut, your DNA and every other part of the body, and it can kill you.

4.

Eating a healthy plant-based diet to ensure gut and mental health, practising good sleep hygiene to ensure sufficient sound sleep, practising mindfulness and avoiding environmental toxins all contribute to stress relief.

5.

Get some sleep. Prioritise it. Practise good sleep hygiene: cool, dark, quiet room. Don't eat within 2-3 hours before bed and stay away from stimulants after noon. Have a bedtime routine and stick to it most of the time. See Carmel Harrington's "The Sleep Diet" in the bibliography for more great information, or go to the Eating Upside Down website.

CHAPTER 9

ANTIBIOTICS AND YOUR HEALTH

During his active 60-year, top-flight medical career Emeritus professor Stig Bengmark has repeatedly called for fewer antibiotics to be used during surgery. Twenty years as head surgeon at the University Hospital in Lund, Sweden, gave him a strong platform to justify his belief that although antibiotics are essential medicines, their overuse is problematic for the health of the wider, international community.

In a brilliant observation he noted that the epicentre for obesity in the United States of America was located around the Southern states like Alabama, Mississippi and Louisiana. He also noted that the highest use of antibiotics was also in this area. He proceeded to compare the two sets of statistics for the rest of the US and a clear pattern emerged: the states with the highest rates of antibiotic use were also the states with the highest levels of obesity. He also noted that countries such as his homeland of Sweden, where antibiotic use was lower than the US, actually had lower rates of obesity. Could this be a coincidence? Hardly. In a compelling argument he concluded that the use of antibiotics could be correlated with the incidence of obesity. Why should this be so?

I DON'T KNOW HOW TO LOVE YOU – serenading antibiotics

The discovery of antibiotics early last century and the subsequent life-saving use of these medicines was, no doubt, one of the greatest breakthroughs in medical science - ever. For all of human history deaths from infections culled the human race without fear or favour for race, gender or pedigree. Even Alexander The Great is believed to have died from malaria or typhoid. With the advent of antibiotics we could save people from sepsis, syphilis and other potentially lethal infections.

Early in the history of antibiotic use it was noted that livestock dosed with antibiotics tended to gain weight faster than those that weren't. Clearly there was a relationship between antibiotics and weight gain. Very soon, it became common practice for livestock breeders to include antibiotics in their livestock feed to ensure that their beasts grew faster, went to market sooner and weighed more when they did so. This meant dollars in the bank and it was cost effective, so the practise continued. What was the mechanism behind this intriguing fact? And what were the consequences?

THE ANTI PART OF ANTIBIOTICS

Pretty much everyone who has taken antibiotics will have experienced the side effects of their use such as bloating, thrush, jock itch, tinea or bowel discomfort. Some people are actually allergic to these medicines. My mother, for example, was allergic to penicillin – she used to come out in a terrible rash. I cannot tolerate Keflex, which makes me violently ill, but if you research the effects of antibiotics there is a whole slew of nasty side effects, and vomiting is only mild compared to some of the others.

According to Drugs.com the side effects of antibiotics might include diarrhea, nausea, vomiting, abdominal pain and a real villain called *Clostridium difficile*, which can kill you if treatment fails. Doctors are advised to keep an eye out for allergies, genital and urinary tract infections, fatigue, and changes in the blood, the skin, kidneys and liver. When you look back on this list and then cross-reference it with information about leaky gut, you will discover, perhaps not surprisingly, that destroying your gut microbes with antibiotics can have some heavyweight consequences.

So antibiotics, although widely used and generally thought of as harmless except to the bacteria they are meant to kill, are not without risk. They are dressed to kill and that's what they do. They really are the heavy artillery in the battle against germs. There are various kinds of antibiotics and some will only work on the microbes that cause specific ailments: an antibiotic for a lung infection may not work for a urinary tract infection, for example, because the microbes they kill are not the cause of both infections. Then there are the broad-spectrum antibiotics, such as tetracyclines, which have a slash and burn mentality. They can kill battalions of microbes, but because they are not targeted they are more ruthless and leave heavy casualties – the gut being ground zero. Tetracyclines have even been implicated in starting autoimmune disease and combinations of antibiotics have a similar effect. So even though we love antibiotics for their life-saving properties, we have to use them carefully, and only when absolutely necessary.

Many patients need to be treated with multiple courses of antibiotics over long periods of times – months and sometimes even years! A trial on women evidenced how the devastation of protective gut flora during prolonged antibiotic treatment can massively increase the risk of suffering heart attack or stroke. This was put down to increased inflammation and narrowing of the blood vessels via a compromised gut.

SWEET CHILD OF MINE – saving baby

Babies come into this world with an immunological halo bestowed on them courtesy of their mother's birth canal. It is Mother Nature's way of protecting the newborn from the onslaught of germs that saturate the biosphere. Being born by caesarean section bypasses this carefully orchestrated procedure and leaves the baby wide open to whatever germs are in their environment. In fact, Caesar babies succumb to infections and tend to be overweight more often than children of natural birth. Experts in the field estimate that children given antibiotics before the age of 6 months put on 22 per cent more weight than a child not given antibiotics and they have a much greater chance of becoming obese within 3 years.

According to Alanna Collen in her book '10% Human' about half of women giving birth in the US are treated with antibiotics *in case* their baby gets strep. The babies are born with antibiotic exposure. To some, such pre-emptive measures may seem a wise precaution but the chances are good that the baby won't get strep either, so destroying the microbiome that comprises a large part of the baby's immune system would seem to be counter productive – even stupid – especially given what we now know about antibiotic resistance. It's yet another case of 'too much of a good thing is still too much'.

Nature's other plan for baby was that it should be fed breast milk. Yes, there is the bonding issue that should also persuade mothers to breast feed if possible, but equally important is the nutrition provided by a mother's milk, which contains oligosaccharides. These substances encourage good bacteria to set up shop in the baby's intestine. The microbes then produce short-chain-fatty acids such as butyrate, which make the gut leak-proof and help prime the immune system. If you remove the basic building blocks of babyhood then the child will be burdened from the beginning. It is becoming standard practise to swab a caesarean baby with its mother's vaginal microbes immediately after birth, and that is a good thing. Some caesarean sections are unavoidable and some of the best-intentioned mothers are unable to breast-feed, but if given the choice, it would be wise to proceed as nature intended: it's an all-inclusive package deal.

EYES WIDE OPEN – know what you're doing with antibiotics

There is barely a person in the Western hemisphere that has not been given antibiotics at some stage. The antibiotic treatment will have impacted the microbiome and maybe even caused problems for the majority of people. This is not to imply in any way that we should never take them! But there are some hacks that will make the impact more bearable and less problematic.

A plant-based diet that supports your immune system can help you fight off disease and minimise the effects of antibiotics, should you need them. According to geneticist Dr Craig Hassan of Monash University in Melbourne, 'Evidence suggests that not only antibiotics, but a high-fat, low-fibre diet changes the balance of bacteria in the gut in such a way as to promote inflammation'. To counter the effect of the antibiotics on gene expression that leads to inflammation and allergic reactions he recommends a diet containing lower amounts of fats combined with high fibre. In other words, lots of plant food and little or no meat or animal products of any kind.

CAN WE GET A TAKE-AWAY?

1.

Antibiotics have an up side and a down side. Used properly for bacterial infections they can be life saving. Used poorly for non-bacterial infections, fattening livestock and to prevent improbable infections, causes actual body and environmental harm.

2.

Overuse of antibiotics in pregnant women and children under 2 years of age can degrade children's guts and leave them open to autism and other problems when given vaccines or if they catch a viral infection from the environment.

3.

The Western diet, which is high in fat and low in fibre degrades the immune system by impairing the gut. It leaves the body open to attack by all manner of micro invaders. Allergies, food sensitivities and autoimmune diseases as well as mental ill health can all take a hold after antibiotic use.

CHAPTER 10

YOUR HORMONES AND YOUR WEIGHT

When people see a fat person they usually think that he or she is lazy or overeats, or both. Rarely, if ever, would it cross their minds that the person is suffering a hormonal imbalance. Yet hormones play a crucial role in maintaining a healthy weight. For me it was PCOS and thyroid, and I will concentrate on these because this is my story, but there are other syndromes caused by an endocrine system that is out of whack. If you believe that you've tried every diet and exercise regime in the book without success, then it's probably time to consider whether a hormonal imbalance is making you sick and fat.

POLYCYSTIC WHAT? - What is PCOS and what causes it?

Polycystic Ovarian Syndrome is a disorder that affects 12 to 18 per cent of women and in some indigenous communities it's even more: that's about one-in-five women. That's a lot.

It has many tell tale signs, most of which are put down to some poor genetic lottery or gluttony, but in reality this syndrome can have serious effects on health if the symptoms are not recognised for what they are and treated accordingly. No, men won't have to worry about this section of the book if they are looking for answers to their own problems, but most will find it useful, because their wives and partners may well suffer from this.

PCOS SYMPTOMS

PCOS can cause irregular periods. It messes with the sex hormones, especially the androgen balance. It can cause hair loss especially in the form of male pattern baldness. Coarse or excess hair, problems with fertility and weight gain, not to mention dry, lifeless and cracking skin are other common symptoms. To make matters worse these symptoms are accompanied by anxiety and depression. It can become a negative cycle of self-defeat. It's PMS on steroids and then some. Symptoms can mimic other illnesses, such as type 2 diabetes, so not surprisingly it can also cause acne and the darkened skin patches that are indicative of insulin resistance and diabetes.

As mentioned earlier, I was on the brink of PCOS disaster, and only by sheer luck was my normal gynaecologist on holiday forcing me to change doctors. Fortunately the second doctor recognized the symptoms for what they were and sent me to have surgery in the nick of time. If any of the symptoms mentioned here sound like you, then it's a good idea to have a doctor check you out.

PCOS TREATMENT

PCOS can be treated with various prescription drugs, but this is rarely a satisfactory solution. Because the underlying cause is hormonal imbalance, the best way to overcome PCOS is to get to the root cause. This will involve blood tests and scans to be sure of the diagnosis, but don't let it come to the point where you have to have an operation to remove an ovary before you get that diagnosis!

Production and use of insulin in the body is impaired in women who have PCOS. Because of this, many of the symptoms and treatments are the same as for type 2 diabetes. Metformin is a drug commonly used to treat PCOS. I took it for about three years and even though I eventually realised it wasn't making any difference to my condition I kept on using it, blindly believing that the doctor knew best. It was a pharmacist who asked me how I was coping with the side effects of Metformin that made me sit up and take notice. Which side effects did she mean? The tendency to sudden eruption of loose stools was first off the rank. I realised that this had been plaguing me but didn't know it was because of the Metformin. Once I stopped using it, the horrendous inconvenience of this particular side effect disappeared. Now that was a relief! Stopping the medication proved my observation that it wasn't making any difference. My blood work remained constant. Only once I changed my diet to low-GI vegan did things start to improve. Please note that it is not advisable to quit any prescription medication without first consulting your G.P.

High levels of insulin can stimulate the ovaries and make them produce excess amounts of androgens – the male hormones. It is thought that excess androgens such as testosterone can stop the ovaries releasing an egg, and lowered fertility is the result. There is a nasty sidebar to this phenomenon: endometrial cancer.

During a woman's cycle a hormone called Luteinising Hormone (so called because of its yellow colour) is released. Women with PCOS can have high levels of this hormone and may therefore be at risk of miscarriage. In her book "PCOS Diet Book" Collette Harris reveals that 80 per cent of women who have recurring miscarriages have been identified as having polycystic ovaries. Anything you can do to manage this syndrome can also help improve your fertility and maintain your reproductive health.

PCOS can be brought on by leaky gut caused by a diet high in carbs, especially wheat and its associated gluten. The syndrome can be devilishly nasty for overall health as it can thwart the most sincere attempts at regulating diet. A vegetable-based diet helps sufferers hurdle obstacles that would otherwise be insurmountable if they continued eating a diet high in processed carbs.

Eating well and avoiding very specific foods is important. In fact, the main theme of this book is brought home once again: food is your medicine.

Now, of course you can keep eating the way you always have, but you will only perpetuate the problem. A permanent change of lifestyle rather than a short-term diet is the key to success for people with PCOS.

What else can you do about it? Well, a tip from Colette Harris that struck a chord with me was to avoid eating too much soy. It is an endocrine disruptor, which means that it tends to mimic hormones in the body, particularly oestrogen. It can contribute to hair loss, which is already problematic for women with PCOS.

You might think that avoiding soy products could be a hard thing for a vegan, but there are so many other sources of protein out there that I just didn't miss it. There is of course seitan, which is based on wheat protein and if you have no problems with wheat or gluten it is a great alternative. Then there are the mycoproteins, based on mushrooms. Delicious, gluten and soy free, these products make the life of a vegan easy and they're tasty as well. There are alternatives to soy milk and soy yoghurt such as coconut milk and yoghurt, almond milk (my preference), rice and oat milk.

Veganism is fast becoming a lifestyle choice for increasing numbers of people, and as the trend grows so does the range of vegan products. Of course, you really can't beat the simplicity of vegetables, fruits and nuts as basic nourishment, but if your creativity fails you or you just want to try something different now and then, there is an ever-expanding range of products available to the vegan consumer. Remember, you can be an unhealthy vegan. If you continue to eat lots of processed foods and sugar-laden treats, your microbiome won't be much better than when you weren't vegan. If you eat a vegan diet that includes high Glycaemic Index foods on a regular basis, you shouldn't expect much of an improvement in your weight or general health.

There is a very close link between PCOS and diseases related to insulin impairment such as pre-diabetes (sometimes known as metabolic disorder or Syndrome X) and type 2 diabetes.

Eating a whole-food plant-based diet with few or no processed foods, can help people with any of these conditions.

THYROID

It is my contention that not eliminating wheat from my diet was the reason my weight loss stalled at 92kg (203lb). The plateau was long and arduous so I got myself an appointment with Doctor Sandra Cabot, an internationally known Australian doctor who is often referred to by her moniker 'The Liver Doctor'. Doctor Cabot has a reputation for being a high calibre allopathic doctor (she topped her year in medicine at Adelaide University) and she has an immense knowledge of various alternative medicines. Her accrued wisdom from both sides of the medical tracks helps her diagnose and treat her patients in a more holistic, less mechanistic way. When I met her she reviewed my historical blood work reports and was dismayed that my GP had not seen fit to attend to what she deemed to be a clear case of hypothyroidism (a low functioning thyroid). I was immediately treated for this and the weight began to shift. And that was great. But what had caused my thyroid to malfunction in the first place?

The thyroid gland, situated in the neck and quite obvious in some people as an Adam's Apple, is a tricky bit of machinery. It is so complicated that most GPs and even many endocrinologists have a hard time recognizing and treating the havoc it can cause when it is out of whack. And it doesn't take much to put it off kilter either. If it's underperforming, a doctor might treat you with Thyroxine (T4), which helps your thyroid produce more of the active thyroid hormone T3. However, if the dose is too high it can stop the thyroid from producing any at all and mess up its function completely. It can also cause nodules to grow. How do I know? You guessed it…. Been there done that.

After a sojourn abroad I couldn't get an appointment with Dr Cabot for several months. She had been treating me with a natural form of Thyroxine. As an interim measure I went to my local GP who gave me a synthetic version but at a dose that was way too high for me and I wound up with a non-functioning thyroid. As Doctor Cabot explained to me, too much T4 (natural or synthetic) prevents the thyroid from producing thyroid hormone and the patient ends up with a severely compromised thyroid gland. For me this turned out to be worse than the original problem, because the thyroid gland objected to the overdose and grew nodules, which can turn cancerous and often need to be treated using invasive methods. Not happy.

VIRUSES AND THE 'MEDICAL MEDIUM'

Whenever something goes wrong we like to apportion blame – it helps us get a grip on the situation and makes it easier to deal with. Whether it's in an argument, after a car crash or during a bout of the flu we hear ourselves saying things like, "I know I sent the email, it must have gone down a black hole in cyberspace!" or "I was in the post office and the guy behind me was coughing all over the place, and he didn't even put his hand over his mouth! No wonder I'm sick!"

More and more frequently the blame for many of the main diseases we come up against is being put down to viruses: cytomegalovirus, Epstein Barr Virus (EPV) and a host of others. A friend of mine, Nova, had been very ill – she had lost 10 kilos in a matter of weeks and just couldn't eat, had no energy and felt entirely depleted. Five specialists later she still had no solution - zilch. I took her in hand and made an appointment for her with Dr Sandra Cabot. Over the years Nova had had various infections, but as a teen in tropical Townsville she'd had Ross River Fever. Viruses are renowned for re-emerging years after an initial infection, often in a slightly different manifestation. Chicken pox, for example, comes back as shingles. Suspecting that her latent Ross River Virus had returned, Dr Cabot put Nova on a course of anti-viral supplements including NAC (N-Acetyl-L-Cysteine). Her health steadily improved and she gradually regained her vitality. She now says she has not felt as well since she was in her teens.

A lot of the reasoning behind the idea of latent viruses seems quite sound, especially when it comes to the connection between EPV and thyroid disease. The thyroid is notoriously tricky to treat and often the medications and treatments don't work in a reliable manner. I have an inkling that the self-styled Medical Medium, Anthony William, might well be on to something when he asserts that viruses are the root cause for many ailments.

After reading the Medical Medium book I went to the chemist to buy some Ashwaghanda, one of the supplements he recommends to rid the body of latent viruses. When I asked for it, the chemist became serious and said it was a powerful agent. She googled info on the supplement and advised me to be careful when taking it along with my thyroid medication, as Ashwaghanda often results in thyroid medications needing to be lowered. Why should this be so?

I interpret this as being a thumbs-up for the Medical Medium's contention that thyroid disease has its roots in Epstein Barr virus infection. Hashimoto Disease may well be defined as an autoimmune disease, but what if the immune system is fighting a real invader – EBV, and not the body itself? This seems perfectly plausible. If Ashwaghanda helps rid the body of viruses such as EBV, then thyroid medications may need to be lowered (or even eliminated) just as the chemist explained. You may think this is just a co-incidence, but what if it's not? Food for thought...

FOOD SENSITIVITY

Exposure to radiation or toxic chemicals can cause thyroid disease, but events that cause such exposure are few and far between. Another cause may be food sensitivity. Considering the huge increase in malfunctioning thyroids across the general populace and a corresponding realization that many more people are sensitive to all types of different foods and products, it seems reasonable to speculate that the two might by linked. Research has shown this to actually be the case.

Eating too many grain products like bread and biscuits can be a basic cause of thyroid malfunction. Grains are hard to avoid in the modern diet and when overconsumption of grains is combined with low levels of iodine and selenium, thyroid problems can arise.

IODINE

Iodine deficiency is prime factor in thyroid dysfunction. The soils in Australia, New Zealand and some parts of Northern Europe are notoriously poor in selenium and often in magnesium and zinc too. All of these are essential for proper thyroid function. Certain foods (goitrogens) have an adverse effect on the thyroid. These include most members of the brassica family such as cabbage, broccoli and Brussels sprouts. People with poor thyroid function are advised to avoid such foods, or eat them only when well cooked. Fluorine, chlorine and bromine can compete with iodine for absorption and thereby cause iodine deficiency, which in turn affects thyroid function. On the other hand, too much iodine isn't good for your thyroid either. A water filter that filters out these chemicals is a really useful addition to your thyroid-repair arsenal.

PITUITARY GLAND

If the pituitary gland fails to produce sufficient Thyroid Stimulating Hormone (TSH) then the T4 will not be converted into active T3, which is essential for proper thyroid function. A fatty liver (mostly caused by the overconsumption on carbohydrates, protein or alcohol) also negatively impacts the conversion of T4 to T3. In women, progesterone deficiency can also create havoc with the thyroid.

THYROID NODULES

Thyroid nodules are another complicating factor in thyroid function. It is important for anyone with thyroid nodules to avoid dairy products as milk is designed to make calves grow quickly. This growth promoting effect can cause the nodules to enlarge very quickly resulting in difficulty swallowing and even breathing. A friend's father was hospitalized, unable to draw breath because nodules on his thyroid had rapidly grown and blocked his airway. Some people even choke on their own saliva because the thyroid or the nodules have grown so large.

CHRONIC STRESS

Chronic stress is often a major factor in thyroid dysfunction. Stress hormones such as adrenaline and cortisol negatively impact thyroid hormone regulation. They increase the production of an inactive thyroid hormone called reverse T3 that is needed to convert T4 into T3. If this process doesn't happen properly the thyroid can't do its job. If the level of reverse T3 is too high you may well exhibit the symptoms of a low-functioning thyroid. I cannot emphasise enough how critical it is to get your stress levels under control.

TAKE AWAY TIME

1.

Undiagnosed hormonal problems have a large part to play in obesity. PCOS and thyroid problems are major contributors to being overweight, especially in women.

2.

What you eat can make hormonal problems worse. A diet high in processed carbs such as bread and pasta, can lay the groundwork for PCOS and thyroid problems.

3.

Grains and dairy can antagonise the thyroid and cause it to malfunction. Eliminating these foods from your diet will make a big difference. See books by Dr Sandra Cabot and Dr Sara Gottfried in the bibliography for further information.

4.

Eating foods in the cabbage family such as Brussels sprouts and bok choy can make thyroid problems worse. They are called goitrogens. If you do eat them, make sure they are well cooked.

5.

Get your stress levels under control. Stress has a profound effect on your endocrine system. It can send your hormone profile way off track.

CHAPTER 11

MY THOUGHTS ON WEIGHT, NUTRITION AND HEALTH

While pharmaceutical companies closely guard their industrial secrets from one another in the search for the golden goose of modern medicines – the anti-fat pill – scientists in the area of gut health seem to have come up with answers to some of the most pressing questions relating to obesity. And there's not a pill in sight.

What causes obesity? Why does it afflict some people and not others? What can be done about it?

Throughout this book we have seen that we denizens of the Western world are well aware that our lifestyle and the foods we eat on a regular basis are causing us to become overweight. Even people who don't eat all that much are getting fat. So are people who regularly exercise themselves to exhaustion. Some people are thin on the outside but fat on the inside. So many people are sick.

Modern society expects that there is a pill to cure anything and everything that goes wrong with us. Well, what if the solution was the exact opposite: NOT taking a pill? What if we replaced psychotropic and pain-killing drugs with simple dietary regimes that are not hard, relentless unappealing graft – regimes that become a lifestyle rather than a diet? We could alleviate much of the misery caused by over-consumption in the Western world. Wouldn't that be a cheaper, healthier and more appealing option?

LOVE MAKES THE WORLD GO ROUND – OR NOT.
Lucre, love and the time bandit

Most people want to be healthy. They pay a lot of money to buy supplements, gym memberships and home-delivered meals. But what they really want is a magic potion – an elixir of life – an easy pill to pop with a glass of water so that life can keep going at its same old crazy pace - that same rollercoaster that, although designed for pleasure, actually robs us of the mental space to pursue fulfilling lives. There are plenty of snake oil salesmen out there with their pills and potions and super food additives – you can spot them a mile off wearing their pristine white coats starched so heavily that the coats could stand up and make a presentation without a body inside them. And most of what they're selling us has just as little substance. It's not expensive pills or hours at the gym that are going to make the massive difference in your life: it's what you put in your mouth that counts, because your diet affects every other part of your life, from your DNA up.

Many people think: 'I love cheese. I could never give up cheese', or 'I love steak. I could never give up steak', or they could never give up whatever their culinary Achilles heel is. What if they knew they only crave these things because of what's going on in their gut – that it's not a matter of will power – that they, through optimum nutrition, can control their genomic fate, which in turn can change the quality of their lives for the better?

Eating habits are formed not just by the culture and family you grow up in, although these things are definitely linked, but also by your genes and the flora in your gut. The microbiome, as the microbes in your gut are collectively called, helps determine what foods you like, which of your genes are expressed and how your cells behave. You really are what you eat: foods, drinks and medicines. More to the point, as I've said before, you are what *your microbes* eat and in the human body they outnumber human cells 9 to 1. They've got the sheer weight of numbers on their side in the battle of the bulge.

Although people have been eating foods that can cause metabolic disorders for thousands of years, those foods didn't have the impact that we are seeing now. We are living in an unnatural world; for one thing, we have changed the genetic structure of many staple foods like wheat, corn and soy. Despite reports of famines here and there, food resources are actually much more secure now than at any other time in human history. Until relatively recent times, humans didn't have 24/7 access to voluminous amounts of poorly prepared, highly processed, man-made food-like substances. In the past, getting hold of a meal was much harder and the foods were in a much more natural state than those we can access in our supermarkets. Nowadays, most people can have the food of their choice at any time they want, just because microbes in their gut flex their hunger muscles and stimulate their appetite.

As for our staple crops, they have been changed beyond recognition. And up to a point that probably hasn't been such a bad thing, but things may have gone too far. The wheat from 5000 years ago wouldn't go anywhere near feeding the world with its current population. But now it is bred to be pest resistant, climate tolerant and top heavy in gluten. Unfortunately gluten is a gut antagonist and has been shown to cause gut permeability (leaky gut), which then adversely affects the function of our brains. We pay a huge physical and mental price to have the soft, delectable bread products and cereals that clog our supermarket shelves.

WHAT DOESN'T KILL YOU MAKES YOU SICK OR STRONGER – your choice

Keeping in mind that fully 48 per cent of people die from cardiovascular disease, 22 per cent from cancer and nearly 10 per cent from type 2 diabetes, and knowing what we now do about the contribution of diet and gut health in the progress of these diseases, we really need to take a close look at what we personally are doing to reduce our chances of succumbing to the big-3. We need to ask ourselves if we want to stay our course on the highway to metabolic hell or take that next off ramp. Most people who end up with the most common diseases eat a diet high in animal products and processed seed or grain products, all of which can negatively impact their microbiome and their health in general. There is no way around the huge dietary landslide blocking the road to optimum health: **either you break your poor dietary habits on a permanent basis or they will break you. Your choice.**

The idea of eating healthily isn't just a ruse to prolong life: it's more a case of putting life in your years rather than years in your life. What's the point of having a long life if you can't enjoy it? What if living is more of a burden than a joy? We've all heard of people who eat ultra-healthy diets but who still die from a heart attack or stroke or some other disease, but keep in mind what we learnt in the chapter on genetics – many factors contribute to disease and although disease may be part of life, who wants to be an amputee lying in bed for umpteen years getting bedsores and all manner of putrid infections because of type 2 diabetes? Stroke, Alzheimer's, Chronic Fatigue, MS - they are all diseases we'd rather avoid. And nobody wants a heart attack in the prime of their life, either. So what do we do about this?

I'm not going to beat you over the head with a stick and tell you to become a strict low-GI, whole food, organic vegan. But, like I said at the beginning of the book, and which has been borne out by significant scientific research; a low-GI vegan diet based on whole plant-based foods will put you on the best course to good health, no matter how much life you've got left. 'Plant-based' does not necessarily equate with 'vegan'. Even if you eat vegan most of the time and keep meat for special occasions, you should still reap the substantial benefits of a high vegetable intake. Your diet is kind of like effective interior design: keep the basics to a neutral palate and change up the small things with colours, patterns and style according to season and fashion!

PROTEIN SHMOTEIN – The protein smokescreen and high protein disaster bombs

High protein consumption is associated with increased risk for cancer. Yes, it will build muscle, and keep you fuller for longer after meals but it will also do a number of other things, especially if it is protein from animal products. Initially, any protein consumed over and above immediate needs is converted to glucose and stored as fat, often in the liver and around your internal organs. This can make you fat on the inside even if you look fine on the outside. This internal fat is called visceral fat and it is the kind that affects your metabolism in a bad way leading to diabetes and other metabolic disorders. On top of that it will raise your levels of Insulin-like Growth Factor-1 (IGF-1).

IGF-1 will help you build muscle, as its function is to enable cells to replicate faster. However, this is the very same reason why it's important to avoid having too much of a 'good' thing. When cells replicate, they split into two parts, each containing mirror image DNA. Sometimes, however, spelling mistakes are made when the DNA is being copied and some cells end up with faulty DNA programs. Usually these faulty cells are detected by the immune system and mopped up and disposed of so they can't create havoc. However, if there is too much IGF-1 the cells replicate too quickly and there is no time for the phagocytes (the immune system cells that eat up unwanted cells) to do their house cleaning. The faulty cells can then multiply again and again, get out of control and result in cancer.

Preventing your levels of IGF-1 from peaking or troughing will benefit your gut, brain and muscles, improve your blood sugar levels and bone density. This molecule has a resumé with a list of notable achievements that is not to be sneezed at, but it is important to realise that having an extremely high or extremely low level of IGF-1 isn't good. According to the authors at selfhacked.com 'having either low or high IGF-1 increases risk of dying from all causes.'

The take away message here is to try to find the middle ground. Eating too much protein will move you away from that happy mid point. It has also been shown that protein from plant sources is less likely to cause major movement in the IGF-1 profile. Avoiding large amounts of animal protein and favouring plant proteins in your diet can help you achieve this desirable outcome. As Dr Sandra Cabot said in her book on autoimmune disease, 'Milk contains growth promoting hormones. … Consuming dairy products can raise your blood levels of insulin-like growth factor 1, and higher levels are associated with a raised risk of breast, prostate and colorectal cancer.' Supporting her contention is Doctor T. Colin Campbell, author of 'The China Study' who quite bluntly says, 'every doctor should tell every man with prostate cancer to stop consuming dairy immediately and embrace a *WFPB diet'. *Whole Food Plant Based.

Protein's important. Choose mostly plant proteins, and don't over do it.

LIFE IN THE FAT LANE –
and too many signs pointing in only one direction

So how *do* you get to be 164kg (361lb) if, like me; you're doing the "right thing" with your diet according to the official guidelines as presented in the food pyramid?

The short answer in no particular order is: genetics, gut flora, antibiotics, bad eating habits established in formative years (environment), stress and trauma (epigenetics). These factors all combine to create a perfect storm for ill health.

A few years ago I was in a consultation with Dr Sandra Cabot when she asked me a question that no other doctor had ever asked me before: "Why do you think you put on so much weight?"

I had already explained to her how I was an obese toddler, obese child, obese teen and obese adult. I had also described a photo of me from the dim vaults of time that revealed a 2-year-old child in a bathing suit, sitting on the top of a slippery dip with a gut any heavy beer drinker would have been proud of.

I had to think about it a little while, but after contemplating all the things that I now knew about the mechanics of weight gain and associated ill-health, I replied that I thought a lot of it had to do with growing up on the land. Now many of you will think that I am stupid for saying this, because obviously not every one who grows up on a farming property miles from nowhere ends up being obese (although the statistics might surprise you!).

When I scanned my mental data bank of obesity-causing factors, my mind easily identified the notoriously scandal-plagued bad guy – highly processed carbohydrate. It is certainly true to say that my diet as a child was heavily weighted in favour of this omnipresent baddie. Dressed in a black hat and bearing arms, he rode into town, hitched his horse to my microbiome and never left. He stuck around and caused havoc wherever he went.

When it comes to food, living on the land has it pluses and minuses. One good thing is that you can grow your own food like tomatoes and cabbages in the home paddock garden. Trouble is, in the back blocks of New South Wales the rainfall can be highly variable – not bad for growing grains but you can't rely only on rainfall for growing vegies. Most of the time it is extremely dry. Drought, in fact. El Niño desiccates the land for 7 or 8 years out of ten. My mother was fond of telling the story of how the whole family had one inch of water in the bathtub to bathe in. As the baby of the family apparently I always got to go first, followed by my older brother, then my mother and finally my father, who had been working out in the paddocks all day. Water was scarce most of the time, so although we did manage to grow some fresh produce, most of our food was in the form of dry foods that could be bought and stored: dried fruits, flour, sugar and jams. A small orchard of fruit trees provided enough produce for mum to preserve fruits in sugar water. As a result, our diets revolved around foods that could be prepared from these ingredients; things like, bread, cake, biscuits, date pudding and pies. We had fresh dairy and my father would also slaughter a beast now and then, so we also had plenty of meat. Eating was a pleasure because my mother was a very fine cook and baker – everything she made was delicious!

After contemplating the description I gave of me sitting on the slippery dip Dr Cabot commented that I was probably malnourished and insulin sensitive even at that tender age. She told me that no child is fat like that without being fed the wrong foods. I now look back and realise that our diets can't have been good for us. You only have to look in the family album to see that my brother and I were extremely overweight youngsters. As tiny tots we were both prone to tonsillitis and my mother has told me that we were given antibiotics to treat the infections until we had our tonsils removed. I was 3 at the time. A diet high in processed carbs and regular doses of antibiotics weren't a good combination for our health. In addition to this, recent research has laid the blame for rotten tonsils in the very young squarely at the door of dairy. Removing the tonsils further compounds the negative affects by removing the immune system's first line of defence.

Although lollies and icy poles were rare treats, other forms of simple carbohydrate were consumed in abundance. If we were hungry we were given toast or a sandwich. To this day I consider bread my nemesis. In the late eighties I used to joke that I had a bread addiction. If I had one piece I felt compelled to have another and it was always as if I could never stop craving it. I now understand that these cravings were caused by the microbes that resided in my gut. An imbalance in the intestinal flora is a major contributor to obesity in today's world. Worse still, eating two slices of bread is no different from downing as much sugar as you find in a can of coke or Mars Bar. The body can't tell the difference and reacts accordingly.

As for the malnutrition, who'd have thought? A microbiome in crisis because of antibiotics and a diet of highly processed carbohydrates depletes the body of many vitamins along with the mineral magnesium, which can lead to high blood pressure, neurological impairment, immune diseases and many other problems. On average, we as a society eat more now than at any other time in human history, but it's ironic that excessive food consumption can and does lead to malnutrition.

Never before have governments and authorities weighed in so heavily on the issue of what the populace should and shouldn't eat. In theory, our diets should be the best in history, but the opposite is true. Turning the food pyramid on its head and eating upside down will bring greater health and vitality to your life. Eating a low-GI plant-based diet high in soluble fibre instead of the standard Western diet will keep you really full, stop you from feeling hungry every couple of hours, help you avoid cravings and sugar lows, plus give your gut microbes food that will heal your gut, keep your mood stable and top up your vitamins for optimum nutrition. What's not to like?

HAVE A DRINK ON ME – alcohol has a hyde – an acetaldehyde to be precise

Some say a glass of red wine a day is good for the heart. Others say steer clear of the devil's blood at all costs. One thing we know for sure about alcohol is that too much is not good, especially if consumed in binge-drinking sessions.

Those polyphenol thingies in red wine are really good for you, aren't they? Yes they are. But alcohol is not the only place you'll find resveratrol (one of those much-touted polyphenol thingies!), so if you're not into red wine, don't start drinking it "just because". Ground linseed and many spices like cloves and star anise contain it, as do cocoa and dark chocolate. (Yay!) So you might prefer a curry followed by a few squares of 85% or 90% dark chocolate instead of the red. Or not ☺

We know some good things are lurking in our favourite tipple but what is it that makes alcohol so contentious when it comes to health? Acetaldehyde actually. I know it was on the tip of your tongue, but being an obnoxious character it didn't want to roll off too easily, did it? Of all alcohol's by-products this is the most toxic as it can alter the structure of proteins. And the building blocks of our bodies, DNA, is protein. Acetaldehyde's most notorious crime is to order antibodies to attack the myelin sheath that protects all your nerve cells (brain cells included) and that can eventually manifest as multiple sclerosis. It's a nasty character.

Good, clean, unadulterated water is your best friend for everyday drinking purposes – straight, on ice or with bubbles – all good. For a bit of light relief you might splurge on any number of herbal teas. If you want to lose weight you should be eating your calories, not drinking them. Drinking the occasional freshly squeezed juice containing the full fibre of the fruit or a smoothie with full fruits should be a treat, not a regular feature of your diet. Such drinks might help you lose weight in the short-term, but they can have sinister long-term consequences - the problem being their highly efficient fructose delivery system.

FRUCTOSE – the sneaky illegal nutrient

Yes, it's natural. Yes, it tastes good, but once in your stomach this seemingly innocent nutrient throws its passport overboard and heads straight for the liver instead of immigrating via the intestine where the body counts the number of calories arriving. Once in the liver it sets up a tab at the bar, converts to fat and glycogen and waits to be picked up and taken to cells needing energy. If that doesn't happen straight away, then it is stored in and around the liver and internal organs as visceral fat. So in small amounts fructose doesn't misbehave, but when it gets with a rowdy crowd it drops its guard and goes wild. It may not get nabbed for a first offence but eventually it will cause real strife – fatty liver. It can take years to develop, but in the long term, excess fructose loitering in your system can crash your metabolism, causing syndrome X, type 2 diabetes or other metabolic disorders.

In his book 'Why We Get Fat', Gary Taubes explains that 'consuming fructose is associated with impaired glucose tolerance, insulin resistance, high blood fats and hyper-tension'. David Gillespie, author of 'Sweet Poison' and 'Eat Real Food' tells us that fructose is 'an appetite-hormone disruptor' that messes with leptin and stops the body from knowing when it's had enough to eat. The proof is out there - we have to be careful when we consume this sneaky nutrient. I've yet to see a piece of salient advice on this topic that does not recommend keeping fruit consumption to a maximum of two pieces per day. More than that on a long-term basis and you're asking for trouble. Fruit is not a totally guilt-free food.

TOMBOLA FOR THE TASTE BUDS – eating the unexpected

Back in the day there used to be a lolly made to look like a row of false teeth. For whatever weird reason, they were actually quite popular and they were sold at our school canteen. My mother told me how one day another of the mothers on canteen duty took one of these lollies and loaded it into one of the meat pies that were also for sale. Boy, did that cause a stir when the poor kid who bought the pie bit into it! Stories abound about what actually goes into some fast foods and they can make you feel nauseous: plastic rice, pig fat dairy, choko apple pies, rabbit chicken, ground horse meat from the knacker's yard… and why don't those damned burgers rot?

Not all of those urban myths may be true, but what we do know for sure is that toxins abound in our food supply, and not just in fast food. Planet Earth is riddled with humans – over seven billion of us. The miracles of science have enabled more of us to be born and survive. Science has also helped us manipulate our agricultural practices to feed the multitudes: genetically modified crops, insecticides to stop nature getting our rations before we do, and herbicides that knock competing plant species on the head so that our crops prevail and they don't. All of these practices increase the volume of food available for our use, but they also leave a chemical trail through our bodies like jet trails on a bright blue sunshiny day.

You can't really ever get away from it, not even if you're eating purely organic produce as part of a vegan lifestyle. You can however minimise your exposure. Your microbiome helps you adjust to just about anything you throw at it, but there are some common chemicals that are just plain bad for you, which you should try to avoid at all costs: glyphosate is one and triclosan another. Let's take a look at them.

I'D LIKE A BURGER WITH A SIDE OF TOXIC GLYPHOSATE PLEASE – chock full of it

Remember, the whole purpose of glyphosate is to kill stuff. It is an organophosphate used to kill weeds and broad leaf grasses that compete with crops. Most households keep a ready supply in their garden shed. A modern farm with no glyphosate is not in the profit-making business. To justify the cost of planting their crops, farmers need to increase the yield any way they can, so they need this stuff to stop weeds from plundering essential nutrients from the soil. Then they need to coat crops with artificial nutrients provided by the same companies that supply the weed killer. Like a quiz show slow reveal, you may see a picture emerging here. And there it is! Chemical corporations bless their little corporate socks, have kindly provided genetically mutated crops that resist the poison they created, so now it's OK to spray the whole field and not have to worry about knocking your crop on the head. So very useful. That way the whole field is ready to harvest in one hit. The trouble is that glyphosate is a systemic poison and knows no boundaries. Just ask the bees that try to pollenate these crops. Oh wait – they're dead and dying - from poison.

Spraying the crop and only killing the weeds is masterful, but this poison doesn't stay only in the leaves, it travels through the whole plant. Animals that eat plants sprayed with systemic toxins like glyphosate take the toxic load on board and are especially good at storing the poisons in their fat cells. Milk, butter, cheese, eggs and meat are all contaminated with pesticides, herbicides and antibiotics. If you don't eat these things you lower the toxic load in your body considerably.

TRICLOSAN – the clinically clean can make you clinically sick

Persistent media advertising would have us believe that a germ-free world is absolutely essential for our health. Buy this spray or use this liquid soap and you can sledgehammer those little critters into oblivion! To the disbelief of many, I have to inform you that such a sterile existence may be doing you more harm than good because such an approach reduces the variety of microbes you are exposed to and makes you more, rather than less, vulnerable to microbial attack. Yes, do wash your hands after the toilet, visiting in a hospital and before preparing food, but there's no need to use the equivalent of a nuclear bomb on a lowly band of rag-tag, unarmed immigrants.

Triclosan is a pervasive chemical predominantly found in products that are intended to reduce or prevent bacterial contamination. This is ironic because once it gets into your system it affects your microbiome in a negative way and impairs your ability to fight off major pathogens like *Staphylococcus aureus* (Golden Staph). It also increases the likelihood of allergies. Triclosan is hard to avoid because it's found in products like clothes, furniture and toys. Because we prefer our personal care products to have a reasonably long shelf life it's usually added to things like toothpaste and makeup as well.

Apart from products that hide triclosan from plain sight, some of us choose to spray it on our benches or gym equipment to get rid of those tricky little germs that lie in wait, ready to pounce and make us sick. Fortunately, when it comes to cleaning, research shows that triclosan can't do anything rubbing with soap and water can't achieve. There's not much we can do about the other products except wash new clothes before wearing them and buy organic personal care products when we can.

Now I can hear you saying, "I can't afford that!" And yes, organic items can be more expensive than your everyday supermarket options. It depends on how you prioritise your health in your personal scheme of things. This is not to say that absolutely all you eat and use has to be organic. That's just impractical for the average person. Maybe you could buy fewer clothes or reduce how often you go out for entertainment. For example, the cost of a small beer will cover the price of quality organic soap; a budget shirt will buy you a bottle of organic makeup and a tube of safe toothpaste costs no more than normal, sometimes even less. If you're playing the long game this doesn't seem much to pay. Then of course, some people just don't have access to reduced-chemical products, but remember the aim is to minimise exposure, not avoid it entirely. As for triclosan, it should appear on the ingredients list of any product it is in, making it easier to identify when shopping.

The issue of triclosan becomes more critical for anyone with thyroid problems or sex hormone imbalances. Studies have shown that triclosan stops thyroid hormones from functioning properly. The thyroid is an immensely complicated structure that is easily put out of whack, and any issues with it can lead to severe metabolic disorders and weight gain. Triclosan will strike at the heart of this metabolic powerhouse. Be aware of this when purchasing products that may contain this hormone-disrupting chemical.

THE OMNIPRESENT CANDIDA ALBICANS – a tough little bug-ger

This one's a doosey. If this microbe made the news, its headline would read, 'Benevolent Interloper Commits Treason'. We are on a friendly first-name basis with *Candida albicans* from the moment we pop out into the world. It's only after a few courses of antibiotics and several years on a diet overloaded with highly processed carbs that we realise he has betrayed us.

Candida albicans is a trickster fungus that likes to wear different disguises, too many to mention and discuss here. One moment he'll be a simple little yeast minding his own business, next thing you know he's like the evil, many-headed Hydra, a mythical Greek monster that makes life absolute hell for mere mortals. Where's Hercules when you need him? One thing we know is that it takes a Herculean effort to slay this monster once he comes to dominate your system. There is good cause to make the effort.

Once out of control *Candida albicans* latches onto cells throughout the body (invasive candidiasis) – in the brain, the heart and any other organ you care to name. In hospitals it is estimated that this bug is the fourth leading cause of infection in patients' bloodstreams with a mortality rate of 30 per cent. In your intestine his tendrils actually bore into the gut lining, making it leaky. Yep. Here we go again! *Candida albicans* can cause the same kind of damage to your gut as gluten and the other antagonists we have met on our journey. As such, it can also wreak the same kind of havoc.

Because *Candida albicans* is a yeast, it really likes to feed on simple carbohydrates: sugar, white bread, crackers, buns and so on. Once it has feasted it turns those sugars into alcohol in the body. The intricate web it weaves will leave you gob smacked. If you have too much sugar in your bloodstream such as in PCOS, Syndrome X, pre-diabetes and type 2 diabetes, then this guy will have a field day. When we take antibiotics we kill off a lot of the beneficial microbes in our gut leaving a lot of vacant gut real estate. Ever the opportunist, *Candida albicans* will jostle in and take over wherever possible put down his hydrae roots and start causing mischief. He will demand that you feed him more and more foods that contain simple sugars, so you will crave bread, chips, ice cream and other processed carbohydrate foods. His appetite and demands will be relentless. The only way to deal with this organism is to starve him out of the fortress. Don't feed him any sugars or other fungi, so nothing that contains grains or dairy. This doesn't have to be forever, but it will take a concerted effort to drive him into submission, cuff him and lead him to the dungeon. You will then need to maintain eternal vigilance to make sure the slippery little bug never raises his ugly multi-headed hydrae again.

HOMOCYSTEINE

"He was so health conscious, how could he just drop dead from a heart attack?", they all said. We've all heard of the health nut that just keeled over and stayed that way. It could happen to anybody. I exercised regularly and all my blood work was perfect: perfect sugar, perfect cholesterol, perfect everything – except homocysteine. It was off the chart! Big time.

I had read about it and thought I'd get my levels checked, as heart attacks run in the family. High homocysteine levels indicate an independently high risk for heart attack, no matter how good every other measure of your health might be. My doctor was sceptical but he signed the form and off I trotted to the pathologist. When I went back to the doctor for my results he was in a conciliatory mood. "Thank goodness you had this checked out!" he said.

Homocysteine levels should lie between 4 and 14 – preferably around 8 to 10. Mine was 38!! My doctor had done some research since my previous visit and was armed with a strategy to lower my rocketing levels. It was simple: take some folate and B6. I did. Now my reading is 12. Phew! That was close!

TRAUMA is more likely to be spoken about nowadays than ever before. Ever since the diagnosis of Post Traumatic Stress Disorder was included in the DSM-IV, studies have been conducted that shine a light on the plight of people who have suffered intense psychological damage in theatres of war, natural disasters and other major catastrophes. But trauma is not confined to these areas.

Great psychological harm is done to millions of people in their earliest, formative years. Such trauma is brought on by poverty, family violence, abuse and neglect. Talking about these types of trauma is still taboo and their hidden impact can ruin lives. Such traumas etch self-loathing, insecurity and acute lack of trust into the psyches of affected individuals.

I could write a whole book on this critical aspect of weight loss, but that will be another project. It is, however, important to understand that even if you are doing all the things outlined in this book and you are losing weight, you might come to a place where you simply cannot lose any more, or you may in fact start to gain weight and feel a failure. Why?

No one becomes morbidly obese for no reason. Somewhere deep inside is a traumatised child seeking comfort and solace from a chaotic world. The actual events may be lost or clouded in the mists of time, but they and their affects are still there scraping away at the soul. Some people use, drugs, alcohol, speed or sex to comfort themselves, others use food and other compulsive behaviours. We started doing whatever it was to console ourselves, just so we could survive. It worked. We are still here with our stories and our cracked and jagged trails through life. But it doesn't have to stay this way.

You need to clearly envisage what your life will be like when you reach your goal weight, or you may be in trouble. Fat protected us, kept unwanted attention away and erected a barrier between us and the rest of the world. A security blanket. Even relationships that seem secure may change and be threatened by your weight loss.

Some relationships work because a fat person and their mindset suits the partner's needs. When that changes, so does the relationship. Sometimes for bad, sometimes for good.

It is critical to be aware of this factor. If you need professional help, get it, but also understand that it is not enough to just talk things through and expose secrets that have been locked away in the recesses of your mind. The actual cells of your body must understand that it is now safe to be who you are, otherwise the addiction will remain and thwart your efforts. Working on this aspect of your life is rarely easy. It's not called the "dark night of the soul" for a tabloid headline. It is essential to have support from friends and professionals.

The brain can change – it is plastic. You may like to seek out practitioners in diverse fields such as kinesiology, Feldenkrais and NLP (Neuro Linguistic Programming) to help you through. When you are ready to take on this work, you will find your way to the right people.

A HEADS UP FOR PEOPLE ON VEGAN AND PLANT-BASED DIETS

There are a couple of things it's good to know before you embark on a plant-based diet of any kind. Nutrients short-listed for the award of "Happiest in House" are: Vitamin B12, Vitamin D, Calcium, Iron, EPA and DHA.

VITAMIN B12 is needed in so many different bodily processes that it's not possible to go into them all here, but it is essential to know that vitamin B12 will keep your brain ticking nicely and keep homocysteine levels down. This information is not just for plant-based eaters. Even meat eaters need to take this into consideration. High levels of homocysteine are linked to heart attacks, strokes and damage to the nervous system. If you're getting enough B12 you won't need to worry. The best sources of B12 in a plant-based diet are fortified motherless milks, fortified cereals and supplements.

VITAMIN D is a key player in the body. It not only helps keep bones strong, it also plays a role in DNA methylation and many other processes. Authorities recommend at least 10 minutes of sun exposure around noon, but failing that there are also supplements and foods: mushrooms, tofu, along with fortified soy and almond milk are the main dietary sources for people on a plant-based diet.

CALCIUM is found in leafy greens like kale, mustard greens, broccoli, tofu, almonds, various beans, hempseeds, rice and molasses. In fact, these sources are more useful for the body than dairy products.

IRON is abundant in plants: legumes, soybeans, tofu, tempeh, lima beans, quinoa, brown rice, oatmeal, nuts, pumpkin, squash, Swiss chard and the list goes on. Cooking in cast-iron cookware can also contribute to iron intake. No need to overdo it, though. Too much of a good thing can be a bad thing!

EPA and **DHA** are important for brain function. Eat flaxseeds. Make sure you crush them first. Done!

KINDNESS AND A 'LAGOM' LIFE

What does it mean to be kind? Does it mean caring? Being nice? Lack of boundaries? All these things?

Too often people mistake kindness with weakness. Their mistake.

Kindness isn't just doing the right thing by others. It's much more extensive than that. So many people, especially women, are kind to everyone in their lives except themselves. Being kind to yourself is essential for good physical and mental health. It's about knowing your core values and beliefs and being true to yourself. Being authentically you.

Saying 'yes' to everything that comes your way via work, other commitments or your family only stresses you out. That's the opposite of kindness. Less is more. Obviously a degree of stress management is called for, and the grab bags of mindfulness, meditation, yoga, sleep and good diet are essential to taming the stress serpent.

The crux to curbing stress is the concept of drawing boundaries. This is simpler if you know what you will and won't accept in your life. Know the difference between important and urgent – they are not the same thing and important always gets precedence. Trauma early in life can lead to poor definition of boundaries – you do what you've got to do to survive, whatever harm is impacting you at the time, but it doesn't have to stay that way.

Research by Bessel van der Kolk at Harvard University has shown that women who were abused at an early age often develop extreme niceness as their way of coping and I've no doubt that it also applies to men. Now niceness and kindness are not the same thing, but they are linked and they can both be tempered by identifying and implementing your boundaries. Obesity is a boundary issue as much as anything else. As with everything, it's easier said than done, but taking steps to befriend your body and becoming aware of what your body feels at any given time is essential to physical and mental freedom. Yoga and therapies like Feldenkrais, EMDR and IFS have all been shown to help people struggling with the aftermath of trauma.

The Swedes have a concept called 'lagom' which means something like balanced, just right. It's about not buying, drinking, eating or doing too much of any one particular thing. It's about being kind to yourself and others and to do this you need to draw boundaries. Start by saying what you mean and meaning what you say - just make sure to couch it in terms that are not offensive That's called assertiveness and it's an invaluable skill to have in your interpersonal arsenal because it helps you find that precious middle 'lagom' ground. Importantly it also helps you avoid those painful win-lose scenarios that nobody benefits from (see the 'Eating Upside Down' blog for suggestions on how to do this). The British actor Miriam Margolyes is masterful in this art. You can see her in action in her "Miriam's Big American Adventure" television special.

Kindness needs to be extended to our co-creatures and our planet too. Everything we do, say, think and feel impacts our world. Be mindful.

ONWARD AND UPWARD –
Caesar and the Romans did win, didn't they?

Yes, Caesar prevailed. Our world has a lot to thank him and the Romans for: paved roads, effective law and administration and a host of other civilising influences. He didn't conquer half the known world by lying back on a divan eating grapes and being fanned by slaves nine months of the year. Leave that to Nero. Caesar knew what he wanted: fame and influence. He knew how to get it: be smart, look after your men and watch your back (although that last one did get him in the end!) The same tactics for success can be used if you want to slay your metabolic demons and gain control of your own life.

If you are not in such good shape, whether you are obese, have a chronic disease or just don't feel you are in control of life, you need to take a step back, evaluate and make plans. What is your goal? Write it down. How are you going to get there? List your strategies and make contingency plans. For many people this will mean deciding to do something about their daily eating, thinking and exercise habits. Obesity and chronic disease don't pop in one morning for a quick breakfast and then go on their merry way. They turn up at every meal for years on end. Getting rid of the unwanted guest will take some effort, but eventually you'll be able to have your morning coffee in peace. But you have to keep working the plan – it'd be disappointing to let yourself go back to the way you were.

After 10 years I have managed to maintain weight loss. Constant vigilance backed by an army of supportive tactics: a good diet, regular exercise, reduced medication and an on-going effort to lower stress levels, have helped me along the way. Why would I or anyone else want to take a U-turn back to metabolic oblivion anyway? Like Caesar, don't lie down on the job; look after your microbes and be ever vigilant. Actually, you might like to show Caesar how that last trick's done.

Remember: "Nothing works unless you do" and as Will Rogers said, "Even if you're on the right track you'll get run over if you just sit there".

TAKE AWAY TIME.....

1.
Modern eating and lifestyles have taken us away from the foods and practises that kept humans healthy throughout the annals of time. Eating a diet full of natural, unprocessed, whole foods, mostly plants, is essential for optimum health.

2.

If you are overweight or obese and you believe your life could be better if you weren't, then you will need to change what you do. Permanently. Going on a diet, losing weight and then going back to your old ways only leads to yo-yo dieting which can be very dangerous.

3.

Most people deal best with change if it is done slowly, in mini steps. This is not true for all people, but if you are someone who tells themselves, "I could never do this or I could never do that" then it will probably be the best approach for you. When making changes, if you fall off the wagon, forget it and just hop back on!

4.

Don't get caught up in the high-protein fanaticism so prevalent nowadays. Too much protein, especially from animal sources, is a bad thing. Eating an equivalent amount of plant protein will not raise your IGF-1 (cancer-causing) levels like animal protein will. There is plenty of protein in plants.

5.

Candida is a nasty microbe. Do everything you can to ensure that you keep it under control in your body.

6.

Eat healthy fats from cold-pressed nut and fruit sources.

7.

Keep alcohol consumption under control. You need to control it rather than letting it control you. Keep the big health picture in mind before you overindulge; remember your gut microbes prefer as little as possible.

8.

Limit your exposure to environmental toxins and chemicals, not just in your home and workplace, but also in your personal care products. They have a tendency to hijack your health in unexpected ways and with negative consequences.

9.
Cover all nutritional bases. Make sure you have sufficient levels of vitamins B12 and D, Calcium, Iron, EPA and DHA.

10.
Get your homocysteine levels checked – even if you're healthy.

11.
Until conclusively proven otherwise, we can say that we only have one life. How we live our life is our choice. Eating a clean, whole food, plant-based diet will give you a firm foundation for living a full life. Eating healthily is about putting life in your years rather than years in your life – although that might happen too. Be kind to yourself, others, the planet and our co-creatures. Remember, animals only get one life too. Before you dig into your next meal think about what it means to take their life for your enjoyment.

GLOSSARY

A

acetate – a substance made from acetic acid (vinegar).

acetaldehyde *[asset-il-dee-hide]* – a compound made in the liver when alcohol is consumed (responsible for hangovers).

acute – severe pain that comes on suddenly.

adipose – describes tissues that contain fat.

adrenaline – a stress hormone secreted by the adrenal glands that causes the heart to beat faster.

Akkermansia munciniphilia – a gut bacteria that helps keep the gut healthy.

ALA (Alpha linolenic acid) – an Omega 3 fatty acid that has to be consumed as part of the diet.

allopathic – treating disease using medicines that have different effects from the disease being treated (the opposite from homeopathic).

allostatic load - the accumulated wear and tear on the body due to stress.

Alzheimer's disease – a form of dementia causing memory failure and disorientation.

androgen – a steroid hormone that causes male characteristics.

aneurysm *[an-you-rism]* – permanent stretching or swelling of a blood vessel wall that can cause it to burst.

antibiotic – a medicine used to stop the growth of bacteria in the body.

antibody – fights against foreign bodies that enter the bloodstream as part of an immune response.

antioxidant – oxygen causes the body to produce free radicals that damage cells. Antioxidants inhibit this process.

artheriosclerosis *[ar-teerio-skler-osis]*– thickening and hardening of blood vessel walls.

arthritis – painful inflammation of the joints.

autism – a condition marked by limited responses to other people and the outside world often with restricted behaviour patterns and limited speech development.

autoimmune disease – disease that arises when the body produces antibodies that attack the body's own cells as part of an immune response

autophagy *[aw-tOff-a-gee]*– the process whereby the body breaks down unnecessary and dysfunctional cells to eliminate or reuse them.

B
B-lymphocyte – a type of white blood cell that is part of the immune system. It produces antibodies that attack invading bacteria, viruses and toxins.

bacteria – microscopic, single-celled organisms that can promote health or cause illness in the body.

Bacteroidetes *[bakter-oy-deet-eez]* – a bacterium that has a symbiotic (helpful) function in the body.

BDNF (Brain-derived Neurotropic Factor) – a protein that encourages growth of neurons in the brain. Important for long-term memory.

beta casomorphin-7 – a naturally occurring product of cow's milk with morphine-like properties that causes allergic reactions.

biotin – a B-complex vitamin essential for the metabolism of fats. Also called vitamin H.

BMI (Body Mass Index) – a measure of whether a person's body is under- or overweight. Calculated by dividing weight in kilograms by the height in metres squared. E.g. 70kg ÷ (1.78 x 1.78) = BMI 22

botulism – a rare and fatal illness caused by the *Clostridium botulinum* bacterium.

BRCA-1 – a human tumour suppressor gene that plays a role in breast cancer.

butyrate *[byoo-ter-ate]* – a substance derived from butyric acid which is found in butter.

C

calcium – a chalky grey chemical element essential in the body for bone strength and other functions.

calorie – a unit used to measure how much energy is in a food.

candida – a yeast-like fungus.

Candida albicans – see Candida.

candidiasis – a condition caused when there are too many Candida albicans fungi in the body that leads to yeast infections like thrush and tinea.

carbohydrate – a compound that can be broken down in the body to release sugars, starches and the like.

carotenoid – a natural red or yellow colouring in foods – related to vitamin A.

casomorphin – a milk protein that has morphine-like effects on the body. It has links to autism, schizophrenia and other disorders.

CFS (Chronic Fatigue Syndrome) – a medical condition that causes fever, aching and prolonged tiredness and depression.

choline – an essential vitamin-like nutrient that is water-soluble. Found in plants.

chronic – long-lasting or lingering.

Chronic Fatigue Syndrome – see CFS. A medical condition that causes fever, aching and prolonged tiredness and depression.

chyme *[kyme]* – the partly digested food that leaves the stomach and enters the small intestine.

Clostridium difficile – (also known as ***C. diff***) a bacteria that causes disease such as Irritable Bowl Syndrome and food poisoning.

coeliac disease (also spelt celiac) – an autoimmune disease caused by gluten in which the gut lining is damaged.

Corticotropin Releasing Factor (CRF) – a hormone involved in the immune response associated with Alzheimer's Disease and major depression.

cortisol (hydrocortisone) – a hormone used to treat inflammatory and allergic conditions.

CRF – see Corticotropin Releasing Factor.

Crohn's Disease – a disease that causes inflammation and ulceration of the bowel. It causes fever, diarrhea and cramping.

CSIRO - (Commonwealth Scientific and Industrial Research Organisation) based in Australia.

cytokine *[site-o-kyne]* – protein that carries signals between cells. Cytokines include interferons, interleukins and other tumour-killing factors.

cytomegalovirus *[site-o-mega-lo-virus]* – a virus in the herpes family.

D

defensins – proteins in the immune system that help kill bacteria, fungi and viruses.

dementia – chronic mental and emotional degeneration causing loss of memory.

DHA (docosahexaenoic acid) – an omega-3 fatty acid found in the brain, skin and retina.

DNA (deoxyribonucleic acid) – the carrier of genetic information passed on from parents to offspring.

docosahexaenoic acid (see DHA).

dopamine – a neurotransmitter chemical that affects the brain's perception of pleasure.

dysbiosis *[dis-by-oh-sis]* – an imbalance of microbes in the gut where pathogenic (bad) microbes cause negative symptoms.

E

E171 – is a food additive used as a whitening agent.

E. coli (Escherichia coli) *[esher-rikkia co-lye]* – a bacterium found in the lower intestine. Many types are harmless but some can cause serious food poisoning.

eczema *[x-ma]* – a non-infectious inflammation of the skin. Often itchy.

EMDR – Eye Movement Desensitisation and Reprocessing. A form of psychotherapy.

endocrine – anything relating to glands and their secretions such as hormones.

endocrine disruptor – a substance that interferes with the proper function of glands and hormones e.g. some foods, plastics and chemicals.

endocrinologist – a medical expert in the function of glands and their secretions.

endometrial cancer – cancer of the lining of the uterus.

endometriosis – a disorder in which tissue that normally lines the uterus grows outside the uterus.

endorphin blockers – drugs such as naltrexone that prevent the body from responding to opioid drugs like morphine.

endotoxins – poisons that are released by bacteria when they die.

ENS (Enteric Nervous System) – the major nerve connection between the brain and the intestines.

Enteric Nervous System (see ENS).

enzyme – a chemical that helps biochemical actions in the body e.g. digestion.

epidemiological study – a scientific study of how disease arises and is transmitted in populations.

epigenetics – the biology of how the environment influences the expression of genes.

epithelium – the thin outer layer of the skin, intestine and blood vessels.

Epstein Barr Virus (EBV) - a herpes virus that causes glandular fever (mononucleosis).

estrogen (also spelt oestrogen) – the main female sex hormone.

F

fecal transplant (also spelt **faecal** and alternatively known as a transpoosition) – putting faeces from one person into another to improve the balance of microbes.

Feldenkrais – a therapy that helps reorganise connections between the mind and body to achieve wholeness in movement and psychological state.

ferulic acid – a compound that helps strengthen cell walls.

fibroid – a tumour containing fibrous tissue especially in the uterus.

Firmicutes – bacteria that have a negative impact. They release toxins, are hard to kill and they cause the body to absorb more energy from food.

folate – a chemical derived from folic acid. Essential for proper development of the foetus.

formaldehyde *[for-mal-der-hide]* – a chemical used to preserve tissue and make plastics.

fructose *[frook-toze]* – a sugar found in fruit.

fungus / fungi – organisms that grow by feeding on other organisms e.g. mushrooms, moulds and yeasts.

G
G-protein coupled receptor 43 – recognises short chain fatty acids and plays a role in obesity.

GABA (gamma-Aminobutyric-acid) – a neurotransmitter that reduces excitability in the nervous system. Also responsible for regulating muscle tone.

gamma-Aminobutyric-acid – see GABA above.

GAPS – see Gut and Psychology Syndrome below.

gastrointestinal system – the body system comprising the stomach and intestines.

gene – part of the chromosome passed from parents to offspring that determines characteristics, e.g. eye colour.

Genetically Modified (GM) – a process of selecting genes to ensure an organism produces a desired characteristic, e.g. tolerance to frost.

genetics – the science of how traits are inherited.

genome – the complete set of genes for an organism.

ghrelin – a stomach hormone that helps regulate appetite and the use of energy.

GI – Glycaemic Index (see below).

gliadin *[glye-addin]* – a protein in gluten that comes from grains.

gliadimorphin *[glye-ah-dye-morf-in]* – (also called gluteomorphin) are chemicals from grains that have an effect on the body similar to that of morphine.

gluten – a protein found in wheat, rye, barley, oats and other grains.

gluteomorphin – see gliadimorphin above.

Glycaemic Index (GI) - a scale that tells you how fast a food converts to glucose when eaten. The higher the score the faster it converts to glucose.

GM – see Genetically Modified above.

goitrogen – a substance that changes the function of the thyroid gland e.g. cabbage.

GPR43 - see G-protein coupled receptor 43 above.

Guillain Barré Syndrome – an autoimmune disease that affects the peripheral nervous system and weakens muscles.

Gut and Psychology Syndrome (GAPS) – gut health and the microbiome affect mental health.

H
HDL – see High Density Lipoprotein below.

hedonic – anything related to pleasure.

hedonistic – pleasurable.

high carb – usually means foods that readily convert to glucose in the blood, e.g. white bread, pasta and sugar.

High Density Lipoprotein (HDL) – the so-called 'good' cholesterol.

hormone – a gland secretion that regulates the action of cells or tissues, e.g. testosterone.

hyperthyroidism – a high-functioning thyroid. Speeds up the metabolism.

hypothalamus – part of the brain that controls automatic functions like hunger, temperature and hormonal activity.

hypothyroidism – a low-functioning thyroid. Lowers the metabolic rate.

I
IBS – see Irritable Bowel Syndrome below.

IFS – Internal Family Systems therapy is a psychotherapy that helps integrate a person's sub-personalities and achieve wholeness.

IgE – see Immunoglobulin E below.

IGF-1 – see Insulin-like Growth Factor-1 below.

Immunoglobulin E (IgE) – antibodies in the immune system that are involved in allergic reactions.

insulin – a hormone produced in the pancreas. It plays a key role in glucose metabolism.

Insulin-like Growth Factor-1 – a growth hormone made in the pituitary gland. Helps reproduce and regenerate cells.

interferon – a protein that helps prevent viruses replicating in other cells as part of an immune response.

interleukin – a protein that helps produce inflammation as part of an immune response.

intermittent fast - a dietary regime that restricts the hours during which food is eaten, e.g. 5:2 diet.

Irritable Bowel Syndrome (IBS) – a stress-related condition with recurrent pain and bowel dysfunction.

K

ketone bodies - are molecules produced by the liver from fatty acids during periods of low food intake and restricted carbohydrate diets.

ketogenic – producing ketone bodies. Used to describe a diet rich in fats and low in carbohydrates to regulate the metabolism.

ketosis – a state when the body uses ketone bodies for energy.

L

luteinising hormone – a hormone produced in the pituitary gland that stimulates ovulation in females and creates male hormones (androgens) in males.

M

macronutrient – a type of food, e.g. fat, protein, carbohydrate that make up the bulk of the diet.

macular degeneration – deterioration of the central part of the retina at the back of the eye. Can lead to blindness.

metabolic – anything to do with the metabolism.

metabolic disorder (also called Syndrome X or metabolic syndrome) – a group of conditions that increase the risk of diabetes, stroke and heart disease including obesity, high blood pressure, fatty liver and high blood triglycerides.

metabolism – the chemical processes that occur in the body in order to maintain life.

metabolite – a substance needed for metabolism to function properly.

methionine – an essential amino acid for humans. Also a methyl donor.

methyl donor – an amino acid that plays a role in DNA function.

methylation – a process that changes DNA and switches genes on or off.

Methyltetrahydrofolate-reductase (MTHFR) – a mutation of this gene prevents the body from using folate properly and prevents the body from eliminating toxins.

microbe – usually a single-celled organism that can't be seen by the naked eye. E.g. bacteria, fungi, viruses.

microbiome – the genomes of the microbes that live in our bodies.

microbiota - all of the microorganisms that live in our bodies.

micronutrient – substances needed in tiny amounts for proper functioning of the body, e.g. vitamins and minerals.

microvilli – super tiny projections from the surfaces of cells that line various parts of the body, e.g. the intestine.

Migrating Motor Complex – gut activity that happens between meals to sweep material through the intestine.

molecule – groups of atoms bonded together that have distinctive chemical properties, e.g. alcohol.

mononucleosis (also called Mono, Kissing Disease and Glandular Fever) – a viral infection caused by the Epstein-Barr Virus.

morphine – is a pain reliever made from opium. Considered to be highly addictive.

MS - see Multiple Sclerosis below.

MTHFR - see Methyltetrahydrofolate-reductase above.

Multiple Sclerosis (MS) – An autoimmune disease where the immune system eats away at the protective covering of the nerves.

mycoprotein – a protein made from mushrooms and other fungi.

myelin sheath – a fatty layer that protects nerve cells from damage.

N

Newtonian – refers to the work of Isaac Newton and his classical (pre-quantum) physics.

niacin – also known as vitamin B3.

nutrigenomics – the study of how foods and nutrition impact the expression of genes.

O

obesity – the condition of being very fat and having a BMI above 30.

oesophagus – the tube that goes from mouth to stomach.

oligosaccharide – simple sugars with many functions such as cell recognition and cell binding. They play an important part in the immune system.

Omega-3, Omega-6, Omega-9 – are fatty acids essential for well-being. Omega-3 and omega-6 are not produced by the body and have to be eaten as part of the diet.

organophosphate – are used as insecticides, medications and nerve agents. Can be toxic.

osteoporosis – a condition where bones become weak and brittle.

P

Paleo – refers to the time before historical records (stone age).

Paleo diet – a diet that excludes dairy, grains, processed foods and sugars, legumes, starches and alcohol.

Parasympathetic Nervous System (PNS) - helps the body conserve energy by regulating heart rate, digestive system and gland activity.

Parkinson's Disease – a degenerative brain disorder characterised by shaking and rigid limbs.

pathogen – a microbe that causes disease.

pathogenic – relates to illnesses caused by bacteria, viruses and other microorganisms.

PCOS – see Polycystic Ovarian Syndrome below.

peristalsis – waves of muscle contractions that move food through the digestive system.

pernicious – having a harmful effect usually in a gradual or subtle way.

phagocyte *[faj-oh-site]* – a cell that can kill and clean up other unwanted cells in the body.

phthalate *[thal-ate]* – substances added to plastics to make them more flexible. Also found in personal care products, air scent sprays, furnishings and floor coverings. They are considered toxic and may cause birth defects.

Polycystic Ovarian Syndrome (PCOS) – a set of symptoms due to high levels of male hormones.

polyunsaturated fats – fats that are typically liquid at room temperature but go firm when chilled.

prebiotic – plants that nourish the good bacteria in the intestines.

probiotic – live bacteria and yeasts that are good for health especially the digestive system.

progesterone – a female sex steroid hormone.

protein – molecules made up of amino acids that are essential to all living organisms. They make up structural components of the body such as skin, hair and muscle.

Proteus – a family of bacteria that cause illness in humans. Often found in decaying matter, sewage and faeces.

protozoa – single-celled, microscopic animals such as amoebas and flagellates.

psoriasis – a condition in which skin cells build up, forming scales and itchy, dry patches.

psychotropic – relates to drugs that affect a person's mental state.

S
Salmonella enterica – a bacterium that causes poisoning of the body.

SCFA – see Short Chain Fatty Acid below.

seitan – a meat replacement food made mainly of wheat protein.

selenium – a non-metallic element essential for many functions in the body.

serotonin – a neurotransmitter (brain chemical) that aids positive mood.

Shigella flexneri – a bacterium that causes diarrhea.

Short Chain Fatty Acid (SCFA) – acids produced when dietary fibre is fermented in the colon. Essential for good health.

Sjögren's Syndrome *[sher-grenz]* – an autoimmune disease that causes extreme dryness of the eyes, mouth and skin.

staphylococcus – a bacterium that causes pus formation.

staphylococcus aureus (Golden Staph) – a dangerous bacterium that is difficult to treat with antibiotics. Can cause death.

stem cell – a cell that can give rise to a variety of different cells such as brain cells, liver cells and skin cells.

steroid – a hormone. Mostly sex or adrenal hormones.

stroke – a sudden attack of numbness or weakness caused by bleeding or blockage in the brain.

symbiotic – when two different organisms live together and benefit each other.

Syndrome X – also know as pre-diabetes and metabolic syndrome. A condition where the liver is fatty and blood sugar levels are elevated.

T
T lymphocyte – a type of white blood cell that plays an important role in immunity.

T3 – a thyroid hormone (triiodothyronine) that affects metabolism, body temperature and heart rate.

T4 – see Thyroxine below.

telomere – the end of a chromosome that protects the chromosome from deterioration.

tetanus (Lockjaw) – an infectious disease caused by a microbe (*Clostridium tetani*). It causes the body to spasm violently and become rigid.

thyroid – a gland in the throat. It secretes hormones that regulate metabolism and growth.

Thyroid Stimulating Hormone (TSH or Thyrotropin) – a hormone produced in the pituitary gland. It regulates the productions of thyroid hormones.

Thyroxine (T4) - a thyroid hormone (thyroxine) primarily responsible for regulating metabolism.

TMAO (Trimethylamine N-oxide)– causes cholesterol to deposit in the arteries. TMAO increases after eating foods such as red meat, soy and eggs. High amounts are associated with heart disease.

TOFI (Thin Outside Fat Inside) – a condition where a person is not outwardly overweight but has visceral fat and possibly pre-diabetes.

triclosan – an anti-bacterial agent found in toothpastes, soaps, detergents, toys and cleaning products. It can affect hormone production and their effects on the body.

triglyceride – make up most of the body's fat. High levels are associated with over consumption of carbohydrate and there is a strong link to arteriosclerosis and heart disease.

tryptophan – is an amino acid. It helps produce serotonin.

TSH – see Thyroid Stimulating Hormone above.

Type 1 diabetes – an autoimmune disease where the body destroys its own ability to produce insulin.

Type 2 diabetes – a lifestyle disease that affects the way the body processes blood sugar.

U
umami – a taste in food like the flavour of meat, cheese, Vegemite.

USDA – United States Department of Agriculture

V

vascular – relating to the blood vessels such as veins, arteries and capillaries.

vegan – not eating any foods of animal origin, including eggs and dairy. A plant-based diet.

Very Low Density Lipoprotein (VLDL) – considered a "bad" form of blood fat because it contributes to clogging of the arteries.

virus – a microbe that can multiply in the body, causing disease, e.g. flu, mononucleosis.

visceral fat – fat around the internal organs. It can become metabolically active. Plays a key role in type 2 diabetes.

vitamin – a compound needed in the diet for optimal health. Deficiency can lead to disease.

Vitamin B12 – has to be obtained from the diet. It helps make DNA and red blood cells.

Vitamin D – is actually a hormone. Produced by the body when exposed to sunlight. Needed for many bodily functions including the metabolism of calcium.

Vitamin K2 – involved in blood clotting and helps direct calcium to the skeleton instead of the tissues and arteries where it can lead to arteriosclerosis.

VLDL – see Very Low Density Lipoprotein above.

Z

zinc – a metallic element essential in small amounts for the correct functioning of the body, especially the immune system.

zonulin – a protein that helps the tight junctions in the gut wall stay tight preventing leaky gut.

BIBLIOGRAPHY

AXE Joshua. *9 Candida Symptoms and 3 Steps to Treat Them.* https://draxe. com/candida-symptoms/. 2016. Internet

BERGMAN John. *Stress is the Cause of Every Disease.* drjohnbergman. com. 2017. Internet

BRAND MILLER Jennie, FOSTER-POWELL Kaye, et al. *The G.I. Factor: The Low Glycemic Index Solution.* Sydney, Australia. Hodder. 1996. Print

CABOT Sandra & JASINSKA Margaret. *The Breast Cancer Prevention Guide.* Camden, Australia. WHAS – Women's Health Advisory Service. 2008. Print

CABOT Sandra & JASINSKA Margaret. *Healing Autoimmune Disease: A Plan to Help Your Immune System and Reduce Inflammation.* Camden, Australia. WHAS Women's Health Advisory Service. 2015. Print

CABOT Sandra & JASINSKA Margaret. *Your Thyroid Problems Solved: Holistic Solutions to Heal Your Thyroid.* Camden, Australia. WHAS – Women's health Advisory Service. 2006. Print

CABOT Sandra. *Can't Lose Weight? You Could Have Syndrome X*. Cobbitty, Australia. WHAS (Women's Health Advisory Service). 2001. Print

CABOT Sandra. *Gluten: Is it making you sick or fat?*. Camden, Australia. WHAS Women's Health Advisory Service. 2014. Print

CAMPBELL Colin T & CAMPBELL Thomas M. *The China Study*. Dallas, USA. Ben Bella Books. 2016. Print

CAMPBELL-McBRIDE Natasha. *Gut and Psychology Syndrome: Natural Treatment for Autism, Dyslexia, Depression, Dyspraxia, ADD, ADHD, Schizophrenia*. Rev. Ed. Cambridge, UK. Medinform Publishing. 2016. Print

CHAITOW Leon. *Clear Body Clear Mind: How to be Healthy in a Polluted World*. London, UK. Unwin Paperbacks. 1990. Print

CHOPRA Deepak. *What are Your Hungry For?*. London, UK. Rider (Penguin Random House). 2014. Print

CHRZANOWSKI and MACIA. *Common Food Additive Found to Affect Gut Microbiota*. University of Sydney. sydney.edu.au. Internet

COSTA-ROBERTS Daniel. *Fast Food Kills Gut Bacteria That Can Keep You Slim, Book Claims*. PBS Newshour – The Rundown. NewsHour Productions LLC. 2015. Internet

COLLEN Alanna. *10% Human: How Your Body's Microbes Hold the Key to Health and Happiness,* London, England. Harper Collins Publishers. 2015. Print

DAVIS William. *Wheat Belly*. New York, USA. Rodale (Macmillan). 2011. Print

DIABETES Australia. What Should I Eat? https://www.diabetesaustralia. com.au/what-should-i-eat. 2015. Internet

DOVEY Dana. *Starvation and Epigenetics: DNA Can Hold Onto The Memory Of Starvation For Three Generations, And Now Researchers Know How.* http://www.medicaldaily.com/starvation-and-epigenetics-dna-can-hold-memory-starvation. 2014. Internet

DRUGS.COM. *Antibiotics. Side effects.* 2011. Internet

DUNN Rob. *Everything You Know About Calories Is Wrong.* New York, USA. Scientific American Special Issue Vol. 309 Number 3 p.p. 46 - 49. 2013. Print

EADES Michael and EADES Mary Dan. *Protein Power.* New York, USA. Bantam Books. 1996. Print

EDE Georgia. *Food Fights: Are Vegan Diets Healthier For The Brain?* diagnosisdiet.com. 2017. Internet

ELSHEIKH Mohgah & MURPHY Caroline. *Polycystic Ovary Syndrome.* Oxford, UK. Oxford University Press. 2008. Print

ENDERS Giulia. *Gut: the inside story of our body's most under-rated organ* Originally published in German as *Darm mit Charme* by Ullstein in 2014 English edition: Brunswick, Australia. Scribe. 2015. Print

FOOD STANDARDS Australia and New Zealand. *Acrylamide and food.* http://www.foodstandards.gov.au/consumer/chemicals/acrylamide/Pages/default.aspx. 2016. Internet

FREEDMAN David. *Are Engineered Foods Evil?* New York, USA. Scientific American Special Issue Vol. 309 Number 3 p.p. 70 - 75. 2013. Print

GAWLER Ian. *Peace of Mind: How you can learn to meditate and use the power of your mind.* Sydney, Australia. 2006. Print

GEDGAUDAS Nora. *Primal Fat Burner: Live Longer, Slow Ageing, Super-Power Your Brain and Save Your Life with a High –Fate Low-carb Paleo Diet.* Sydney, Australia. Allen & Unwin. 2017. Print

GILLESPIE David. *Sweet Poison*. Melbourne, Australia. Viking (Penguin Books). 2008. Print

GILLESPIE David. *Eat Real Food: The Only Solution to Permanent Weight Loss and Disease Prevention*. Sydney, Australia. Pan Macmillan. 2015. Print

GILLESPIE David. *Toxic Oil: Why Vegetable Oil Will Kill You & How to Save Yourself*. Melbourne. Viking (Penguin Books). 2012. Print

GLENVILLE Marilyn. *Fat Around the Middle: How to Lose That Bulge – For Good*. London, UK. Kyle Cathie Ltd. 2006. Print

GOTTFIRED Sara. *Younger: The Breakthrough Programme to Reset our Genes and Reverse Ageing*. London, UK. Vermillion (Penguin Random House). 2017. Print

GOTTFRIED Sara. *The Hormone Reset Diet*. New York. Harper Collins. 2015. Print

GREGER Michael. *How Not To Die*. London, UK. Pan Books Macmillan. 2016
First published 2015 by Flatiron Books. Print

HARRINGTON Carmel. The Sleep Diet. Pan. Sydney, Australia. Pan MacMillan. 2012 Print

HARRIS Colette & CHEUNG Theresa. *The PCOS Diet Book: How you can use the nutritional approach to deal with polycystic ovarian syndrome*. London, UK. Thorsons (Harper Collins). 2002. Print

HASSED Craig. *Playing the genetic Hand Life Dealt You*. Melbourne, Australia. Michelle Anderson Publishing. 2014. Print

HELLER Rachael and HELLER Richard. *The Carbohydrate Addict's Diet*. Ringwood, Australia. Signet (Penguin). 2000. First published in Signet by Penguin Books USA 1993. Print

KELLMAN Raphael. *The Microbiome Diet: The Scientifically Proven Way to Restore Your Gut health and Achieve Permanent Weight Loss.* Boston USA. Da Capo Lifelong Books. 2014. Print

KENNY Paul. *The Food Addiction.* New York, USA. Scientific American Special Issue Vol. 309 Number 3 pp 34 -39. 2013. Print

KIM Evelyn. *The Amazing Multimillion-year history of Processed Food.* New York, USA. Scientific American Special Issue Vol. 309 Number 3 p.p. 40 - 45. 2013. Print

KOTZ Deborah. *Eating More Whole Grain Is Worth The Trouble.* Boston, USA. The Boston Globe. 16 January 2015. Internet

LAWRENCE Felicity. *Not on the Label: What really goes into the food on your plate.* London, UK. Penguin Books. 2004. Print

LEAKY GUT SYNDROM.DE. *Leaky Gut Syndrom – der durchl*ässige *Darm.* http://leakygutsyndrom.de/. Internet

LEECH Joe. *MTHFR Mutation, Symptoms and Diet: What You Need To Know.* https://www.dietvsdisease.org>mthfr-mutation. 2017. Internet

LEVINOVITZ Alan. *The Gluten Lie.* Collingwood, Australia. Nero (Schwartz Publishing). 2015. Print

LIPTON Bruce. *The Biology of Belief: Unleashing the Power of Consciousness, Matter and Miracles.* 5th Ed. .... Hay House. 2009. Print

LUDWIG David S & FRIEDMAN Mary. *Always Hungry? Here's Why.* New York, USA. New York Times 15 May 2014. Internet

LUDWIG David S. *Could Your Healthy Diet Make Me Fat?* New York, USA. The New York Times. 28 November 2015. Internet

LUSTIG Robert. *Fat Chance: The Bitter Truth About Sugar.* London, UK. Fourth Estate (Harper Collins). 2013. Print

MATE Gabor. When the body Says No: Exploring the stress-disease connection. Hoboken, USA. John Wiley and Sons. First published in Canada by Alfred Knopf. 2003. Print

MAYER Emeran. *The Mind-Gut Connection: How the Hidden Conversation Within Our Bodies Impacts Our Mood, Our Choices and Our Overall Health,* New York, USA, Harper Collins. 2016. Print

MEARES Ainslie. Relief Without Drugs: The Self-Management of Tension, Anxiety and Pain. Sydney, Australia. Harper/Collins Publishers. 1983. Print

MERCOLA Joseph. *Why Low Cholesterol Is Not Good For You.* http://articles.mercola.com/sites/articles/archive/2008/07/15/why-low-cholesterol-is-not-good-for-you. 2008. Internet

MOSLEY Michael. *Should I Eat Meat?* SBS Television Australia. 25 May 2017. Television.

MOSLEY Michael and SPENCER Mimi. *The Fast Diet: The Simple Secret of Intermittent Fasting.* London, UK. Short Books. 2013. Print

MOSLEY Michael. *The Clever Guts Diet: How to revolutionise your body from the inside out.* Cammeray, Australia. Simon & Schuster. 2017. Print

MOYER Michael. *The Food Issue.* New York, USA. Scientific American Special Issue Vol. 309 Number 3 p.p. 24-29. 2013. Print

NATIONAL Health and Medical Research Council. *Eat for Health.* Australian Dietary Guidelines Summary. 2013. https://www.eatforhealth.gov.au. 2015. Internet

PAUL Sharad P. *The Genetics of Health: Understand Your Genes for Better Health.* Cammeray, Australia. Simon & Schuster. 2017. Print

PERLMUTTER David & LOBERG Kristin. *Brain Maker: The Power of Gut Microbes to Heal and Protect Your Brain – for Life*. London, UK. Yellow Kite (Hodder and Stoughton). 2015 Print

PERLMUTTER David & LOBERG Kristin. *Grain Brain: The Surprising Truth About Wheat, Carbs and Sugar – Your Brain's Silent Killers*. London, UK. Yellow Kite (Hodder and Stoughton). 2014 Print

PERLMUTTER David & LOBERG Kristin. *The Grain Brain Whole Life Plan*. London, UK. Yellow Kite (Hodder & Stoughton). 2016. Print

POLLAN Michael. *In Defence of Food: The Myth of Nutrition and the Pleasures of Eating*. London, UK. Penguin Books, 2009. (First published in the USA by The Penguin Press 2008) Print

PRAXISKLINIK FÜR DIAGNOSTIK UND PRIVATMEDIZIN BORNHEIM. *Auffällige Cholesterinwerte*. http://www.cholesterinspiegel.de/ursachen-fuer-schlecte-cholesterinwerte/. Internet

SAVILL Antoinette and HAMILTON Dawn. *Lose Wheat Lose Weight*. London, UK.
Thorsons (Harper Collins). 2001. Print

SAYER Ji. *How Low Cholesterol Can Harm Your Health*. GreenMedinfo. 2012. Internet

SEARS Barry & LAWREN Bill. *Enter The Zone*. New York, USA. Regan (Harper Collins). 1995. Print

SPECTOR Tim. *The Diet Myth: The Real Science Behind What We Eat*. London, UK. Weidenfeld and Nicolson (Hachette). 2015. Print

STEPHEN Louise. *Eating Ourselves Sick: How modern food is destroying our health*. Sydney, Australia. Pan Macmillan. 2017. Print

STIX Gary. *The Case For Milk Is Going Sour*. New York, USA. Scientific American Special Issue Vol. 309 Number 3 p.20. 2013. Print

TAUBES Gary. *Good Calories Bad Calories*. New York, USA. Alfred A Knopf (Random House). 2007. Print

TAUBES Gary. *Which One Will Make You Fat?* New York, USA. Scientific American Special Issue Vol. 309 Number 3 p.p. 50 - 55. 2013. Print

TEICHOLZ Nina. *The Big Fat Surprise*. New York, USA. Scribe. 2014 This edition Simon and Schuster 2014. Print

WIKIPEDIA. *Insulinähnliche Wachstumfaktoren*. https://de.wikipedia. org-wiki-Insulin%C3%A4hnliche_Wachstumfaktoren. 2016 Internet.

VAN DER KOLK Bessel. *The Body Keeps the Score: Brain, Mind and Body in the Healing of Trauma*. New York, USA. Penguin Books. 2014. Print

WALIA Arjun. *Neuroscientist Shows What Fasting Does To Your Brain and Why Big Pharma Won't Study It*. http://realpharmacy.com/neuroscientist-fasting/. 2015. Internet

WRANGHAM Richard. *The First Cookout*. New York, USA. Scientific American Special Issue Vol. 309 Number 3 p.p. 56 - 59. 2013. Print

ZENTRUM DER GESUNDHEIT. Leaky Gut Syndrom – Ursachen und Therapie. https://www.zentrum-der-gesundheit.de/leaky-gut-syndrom. html. 2016. Internet

ACKNOWLEDGEMENTS

There are many people who have helped me in the preparation of this book. First and foremost I would like to thank my long-time friend and post-grad supervisor Frau Dr Angelika Thiele for putting the idea of this book in my head – never would have thought to do it without your inspiration!

Thank you to Louisa Butler and Norma Odenthal for your invaluable suggestions, proofing, feedback and all-round good-eggness! To Helen Ritchie for your guidance and encouragement. To Karl Schaffarczyk for creating my blog site, solving an incalculable number of technical problems and providing a legal guiding hand. To Sally-Anne Whitten and Di Stacey for guinea-pigging the finished product and giving feedback. Di also took the fabulous 'after' photos and made me look a million bucks while Louise Campbell of Digit Design Studio brought the cover design to life. And lastly, to Scott V Grube for coming up with the brilliant title. I couldn't have done it without you all!

Love Belinda

ABOUT THE AUTHOR

Belinda Butler is an accomplished teacher, writer and musician. Her PhD research in didactics at the Westfälische Wilhelms-Universität in Münster (1988–1991), Germany focused on the role of motivation in teaching and learning. This practical knowledge has underpinned her success in writing, teaching and public speaking.

Her writing opus includes several suites of foreign language textbooks, professional development works and a self-motivation book.

Belinda has spent the last 16 years teaching prisoners with challenging backgrounds at the Tamworth Correctional Centre in New South Wales, Australia. She has helped troubled learners to achieve credible results in reading, writing and maths and many have been inspired to pursue further education upon release.

After her studies in Germany Belinda worked as a teacher, interpreter and translator in Sweden. Most of her work there was medical interpreting and she got to know a whole lot about the cutting edge medical procedures for the cardiac surgery of the time. It was fascinating work and she thrived on it because she got to combine her love of science with her gift for foreign languages.

After returning to Australia Belinda completed a Diploma in Journalism and worked part-time as a journalist at *The Northern Daily Leader* in Tamworth before taking up a full-time teaching position. She is a full member of the Australian Society of Authors and was A/President of the Tamworth chapter of Zonta International.

Belinda has developed a strong reputation for delivering engaging public talks and lectures in Sweden, Germany and Australia. She has participated in Educational symposia and has been interviewed on radio. She writes a blog analogue to her book called "Eating Upside Down" and actively researches in her areas of interest (education, health, nutrition and physics).

Here is a list of her previous publications:

Veganaut – A selection of poems 1980 to 1989 – 2019 Kindle Direct Publishing

Tricks of the Teaching Trade – A Manual for Beginning Teachers of LOTE/ ESL - 2004 Knowledge Books and Software, Brisbane, Australia

Lifemoves - 2004 Knowledge Books and Software, Brisbane, Australia

Bahasa Indonesia - 1998 Sonic Grooves, Bowral, Australia

Visage de Franc -1998 Sonic Grooves, Bowral, Australia

Learning Made Fast and Fun - 1998 Sonic Grooves, Bowral, Australia

Sweden (text and workbook) - 1994 Rebus Publishing, Bowral, Australia

Capisco L'Italiano 1 – 3 (set of text/workbooks in kit form) - 1994 Rebus Publishing, Bowral, Australia

Achieving Proficiency in the Classroom - 1994 Australian Language and Literacy Council

Kapito Deutsch 1 – 10 (set of text/workbooks in kit form) - 1994 Rebus Publishing, Bowral, Australia

INDEX